Recent Results in Cancer Research 67

Fortschritte der Krebsforschung
Progrès dans les recherches sur le cancer

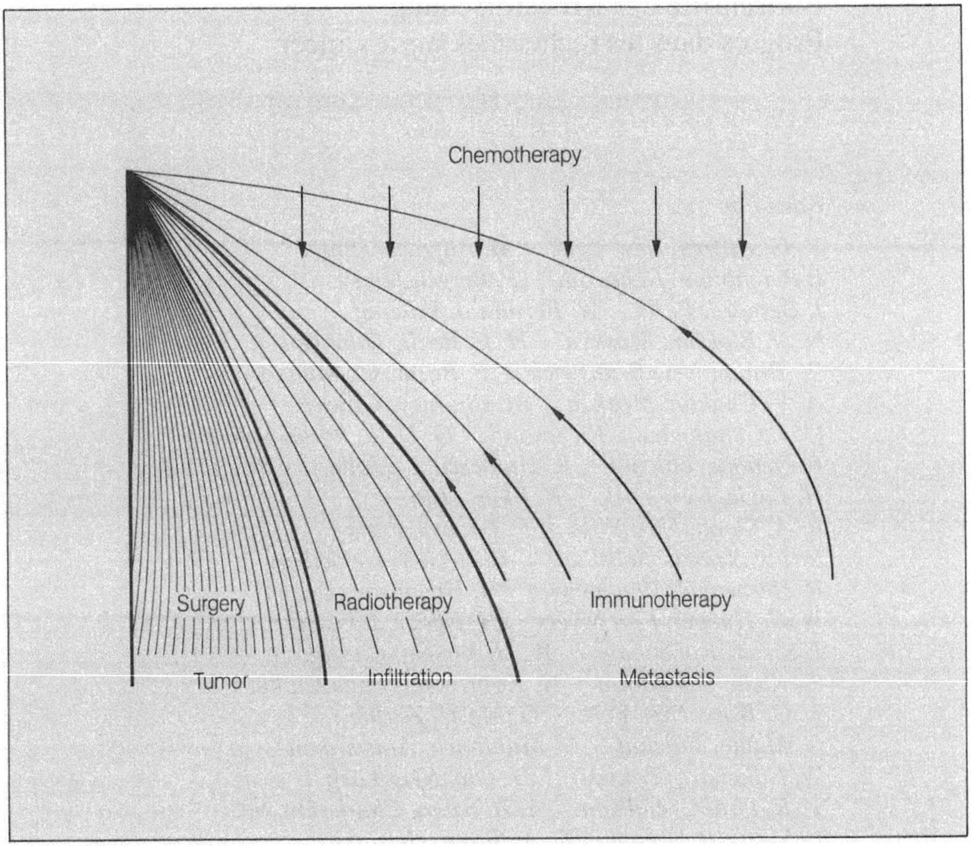
Chemotherapy
Surgery
Radiotherapy
Immunotherapy
Tumor
Infiltration
Metastasis

Adjuvant Therapies and Markers of Post-Surgical Minimal Residual Disease I

Markers and General Problems of Cancer Adjuvant Therapies

Edited by
G. Bonadonna G. Mathé S. E. Salmon

With 64 Figures and 40 Tables

Springer-Verlag
Berlin Heidelberg New York 1979

1978 Annual Plenary Meeting of the European Organization for Research on Treatment of Cancer, Paris, June 1978

Professor Gianni Bonadonna
Istituto Nazionale dei Tumori,
Via Venezian 1
I-20133 Milano

Professor Georges Mathé
Institut de Cancérologie et d'Immunogénétique
Hôpital Paul-Brousse, 14–16, Avenue Paul-Vaillant-Couturier
F-94800 Villejuif

Professor Sydney E. Salmon
University of Arizona Cancer Center
1501 North Campbell Ave.
Tucson, Arizona 85724/USA

Sponsored by Swiss League against Cancer

ISBN-13:978-3-642-81322-1 e-ISBN-13:978-3-642-81320-7
DOI: 10.1007/978-3-642-81320-7

Library of Congress Cataloging in Publication Data. European Organization for Research on Treatment of Cancer. Adjuvant therapies and markers of post-surgical minimal residual disease I & II. (Recent results in cancer research; 67–68) "1978 annual plenary meeting of the European Organization for Research on Treatment of Cancer, Paris, June 1978." "Sponsored by the Swiss League against Cancer." Bibliography: p. Includes index. 1. Cancer-Congresses. 2. Cancer-Surgery-Congresses. 3. Tumor proteins-Congresses. 4. Therapeutics-Congresses. I. Bonadonna, G., 1934 – II. Mathé, Georges, 1922 – III. Salmon, Sydney E. – IV. Schweizerische Nationalliga für Krebsbekämpfung und Krebsforschung. – V. Title. VI. Series. RC261.R35 no. 67-68 [RC270.8] 616.9'94'008s 79-9998 [616.9'94'06]

Softcover reprint of the hardcover 1st edition 1979

2125/3140–543210

Contents

II. Adjuvant Therapies of Post-Surgical Minimal Residual Disease

A. Rational and Experimental Basis of Post-Surgical Residual Therapies

Contents of Volume 68

Adjuvant Therapies and Markers of Post-Surgical Minimal Residual Disease II

List of Participants

V. Adamson, see H. Strander

D. S. Alberts, see S. E. Salmon

W. E. C. Allt, see J. W. Meakin

W. K. Amery, Clinical Department Research Laboratoria, Janssen Pharmaceutica, B-2340 Beerse

J. L. Amiel, Institut Gustave-Roussy, 16 bis, Avenue Paul-Vaillant-Couturier, F-94800 Villejuif

T. Aparisi, see H. Strander

C. Ardiet, see E. Pommatau

R. W. Baldwin, Cancer Research Campaign Laboratories, Univ. Nottingham, Nottingham NG7 2 RD U.K.

B. Banzet, see C. Jacquillat

A. Baron, CMC de Bligny, F-91640 Briis sous Forges

J. Baumann, Président, Académie de Chirurgie, 26, Boulevard Raspail, F-75007 Paris

F. Bayet, see F. Lacour

M. Bayssas, see G. Mathé, (1)

F. A. Beale, see J. W. Meakin

R. Belanger, see T. H. M. Stewart

S. Bellaich, see C. Jacquillat

G. Beretta, see U. Veronesi

X. Y. Bertagna, Dept. Medicine and Cancer Research Center, Vanderbilt University School of Medicine, Nashville, TN 37232/USA

J. C. Bertrand, Service de Biomathématiques, CHU Pitié-Salpétrière, 47, Boulevard de l'Hôpital, F-75634 Paris-Cedex

H. J. G. Bloom, Royal Marsden Hospital and Institute of Cancer Research, London SW3/U.K.

G. R. Blumenschein, see J. U. Gutterman

M. Boiron, Hôpital Saint-Louis, 2 Place du Docteur- A. Fournier F-75010 Paris

G. Bolis, see C. Mangioni

G. Bonadonna, Istituto Nazionale per lo Studio e la Cura dei Tumori, Via Venezian 1, I-20133 Milan

E. Bonmassar, Institute of Pharmacology, University of Perugia, Via del Gioghetto, I-06100 Perugia

C. Brambilla, see G. Bonadonna

V. H. C. Bramwell, Christie Hospital and Holt Radium Institute, Wilmslow Road, Manchester M 20 9BX/U.K.

K. Breur, see E. van der Schueren

R. Brossel, Département de Radiothérapie, Hôpital Tenon, 4, Rue de la Chine, F-75970 Paris-Cedex 20

L. Broström, see H. Strander

M. Bruley-Rosset, Institut de Cancérologie et d'Immunogénétique (ICIG), Hôpital Paul-Brousse, 14–16, Avenue Paul-Vaillant-Couturier, F-94800 Villejuif

M. Brunat-Mentigny, see E. Pommatau

D. Buffe, Institut de Cancérologie et d'Immunogénétique (ICIG), Hôpital Paul-Brousse, 14–16, Avenue Paul-Vaillant-Couturier, F-94800 Villejuif

A. Buge, Clinique Neurologique, Hôpital de la Salpétrière, 83, Boulevard de l'Hôpital, F-75013 Paris

R. D. Bulbrook, Imperial Cancer Research Fund, London/U.K.

M. A. Burgess, see J. U. Gutterman

P. Burtin, Institut de Recherches Scientifiques sur le Cancer (IRSC), CNRS, BP8, F-94800 Villejuif

R. S. Bush, see J. W. Meakin

A. V. Buzdar, see J. U. Gutterman

D. E. Bytell, see S. G. Taylor

K. Cantell, Central Public Health Laboratories, Mannenhemintie 166, SF-00280 Helsinki

P. Cappelaere, Centre Oscar Lambret, F-59000 Lille

R. W. Carey, see S. D. Kaufman

P. Cassell, see J. M. Gilbert

D. Chassagne, Institut Gustave-Roussy, 16 bis, Avenue Paul-Vaillant-Couturier, F-94800 Villejuif

J. L. Chassard, see E. Pommatau

Cl. Chastang, Chu Pitié-Salpétrière, 47, Boulevard de l'Hôpital, F-75634 Paris-Cedex

C. Chenal, Hôpital de la Salpétrière, 83, Boulevard de l'Hôpital, F-75013 Paris

Y. C. Cheng, see E. Mihich

P. Chollet, Centre Jean Perrin, Place Henri-Dunant, F-63000 Clermont-Ferrand

J. Civatte, see C. Jacquillat

R. M. Clark, see J. W. Meakin

P. Clifford, Chester Beatty Research Institute, Royal Marsden Hospital, London SX3 6JJ/U.K.

E. H. Cooper, Unit for Cancer Research, University of Leeds, Leeds LS2 9NL/U.K.

J. F. Cooper, Department of Urology, Southern California Permanente Medical Group, 4955 Sunset Boulevard, Los Angeles, CA 90027, USA

P. Corbett, see B. Richards

G. N. Cornell, see T. B. Grage

E. P. Cortes, Long Island Jewish-Hillside Medical Center, New Hyde Park, New York, NY/USA

J. Cosemans, University of Leuven, B-3000 Leuven

A. B. Cosimi, see S. D. Kaufman

F. Cottenot, see C. Jacquillat

P. Creaven, see E. Mihich

A. Crepeau, see T. H. M. Stewart

A. Crook, see T. H. M. Stewart

M. E. Crowther, see C. N. Hudson

O. M. Curling, see C. N. Hudson

D. Dantchev, see G. Mathé (1)

D. G. Decker, see J. H. Edmonson

H. Deicher, see H. H. Peter

G. Delage, see F. Lacour

M. Delgado, see G. Mathé (1)

L. Denis, EORTC Data Center, Institut Jules Bordet, 1, Rue Heger Bordet, B-1000 Brussels

P. Denoix, Director UICC and Institut Gustave-Roussy, 16 bis, Avenue Paul-Vaillant-Couturier, F-94800 Villejuif

A. Depierre, see L. Israel

M. D'Incacci, see C. Mangioni

J. Domas, see B. Serrou

J. P. Droz, see J. L. Amiel

D. Durand, Fondation Bergonié, 180, Rue Saint-Genès, F-33000 Bordeaux

G. A. Edelstyn, Northern Ireland Centre for Radiotherapy and Oncology, Belfast BT8 8JR/U.K.

J. H. Edmonson, Mayo Clinic, Rochester, MN 55901/USA

S. Einhorn, see H. Strander

H. Ellis, Westminster Hospital, London/U.K.

E. Engelsman, Internal and Radiotherapy Depts., Antoni Van Leeuwenhoek Hospital, The Netherlands Cancer Institute, Plesmanlaan 21, Amsterdam, The Netherlands

E. Eschwege, see J. L. Amiel

A. Fassas, Institut de Cancérologie et d'Immunogénétique (ICIG), Hôpital Paul-Brousse, 14–16, Avenue Paul-Vaillant-Couturier, F-94800 Villejuif

T. R. Fleming, see J. H. Edmonson

I. Florentin, see G. Mathé (1)

F. Fossati-Bellani, see G. Bonadonna

A. Foti, Dept. of Research, Southern California Permanente Medical Group, 4955 Sunset Blvd, Los Angeles, CA 90027/USA

P. Franchimont, Radio-immunoassay Laboratory, CHU Tour de Pathologie, Sart Tilman, B-Liege 1

E. J. Freireich, see J. U. Gutterman

R. W. Frelick, see T. B. Grage

U. Ganzinger, Erste Medizinische Klinik, Universität Wien, Lazarettgasse 14, A-1090 Vienna

J. Gary-Bobo, see B. Serrou

M. Gasparini, see G. Bonadonna

L. Gauci, see B. Serrou

H. Gautier, CMC de Bligny, F-91640 Briis sous Forges

E. A. Gehan, see J. U. Gutterman

A. F. C. Gerristen, see L. M. van Putten

J. M. Gilbert, Wexham Park Hospital, Slough, Middlesex/U.K.

M. A. Gil-Delgado, see G. Mathé (2)

G. R. Giles, University Department of Surgery, Saint James' University Hospital, Leeds LS2 9NL/U.K.

G. Giordano, see S. E. Salmon

R. W. Glashan, see B. Richards

O. Glidewell, Cancer and Leukemia Group B Operation Office Scarsdale, New York, NY 10021/USA

J. C. Goffin, EORTC Cooperative Group, Centre René Goffin, Centre Hospitalier de Tivoli, Avenue Max Buset 34, B-7100 La Louviere

A. Goldin, Division of Cancer Treatment, National Cancer Institute, Bethesda, MD 20014/USA

H. C. Gooszen, Saint Antonius Hospital, Utrecht, The Netherlands

J. Gouveia, see G. Mathé (2)

T. B. Grage, University of Minnesota Hospital, Dept. of Surgery, Box 90 Mayo, Minneapolis, MN 54555/USA

A. A. Green, St. Jude Children's Hospital, 332 North Lauderdale, Memphis, TN 38101/USA

D. Guerin, ChU de Rennes, 2, Rue de l'Hôtel-Dieu, F-35000 Rennes

J. U. Gutterman, Departments of Medicine, Developmental Therapeutics and Biomathematics, University of Texas System Cancer Center, MD Anderson Hospital and Tumor Institute, Houston, TX 77030/USA

K. Hall, see H. Strander

K. E. Halnan, Glasgow Institute of Radiotherapeutics and Oncology, Western Infirmary, Glasgow G11 6NT/U.K.

E. Hamersma, see E. Engelsman

J. E. Harris, see T. H. M. Stewart

M. Hartmann, Urological Department of the Federal Armed Forces Station Hospital, Lesserstraße 180c, D-2000 Hamburg

J. L. Hayard, Imperial Cancer Research Fund, London/U.K.

M. Hayat, see G. Mathé, (1 u. 2)

K. Hellman, Imperial Cancer Research Fund, Lincoln's Inn Fields, London WC2A 3PX/U.K.

J. C. Hendrick, see P. Franchimont

R. Henry, Union Carbide, 4, Place des Etats-Unis, F-94533 Rungis

J. Hermon-Taylor, see G. M. Gilbert

E. M. Hersh, see J. U. Gutterman

R. Heusinkveld, see S. E. Salmon

G. A. Higgins, Department of Surgery, Georgetown University Hospital, and Veterans Administration Hospital, Washington, DC 20007/USA

E. Y. Hilal, Memorial Sloan Kettering Cancer Center, New York, NY 10021/USA

J. Hildebrand, Institut Jules Bordet, 1, Rue Heger-Bordet, B-1000 Brussels

G. J. Hill, see T. B. Grage

Y. Hirshaut, Memorial Sloan Kettering Cancer Center, New York, NY 10021/USA

W. Hirte, see T. H. M. Stewart

B. Hoerni, Fondation Bergonié, 180, Rue Saint-Genès, F-33000 Bordeaux

H. Höffken, see R. W. Baldwin

D. Hoffstetter, Centre Alexis Vautrin, F-54000 Nancy

J. F. Holland, Mount Sinai Hospital School of Medicine, New York, NY 10021/USA

A. Hollingshead, see T. H. M. Stewart

D. Hooper, see T. H. M. Stewart

H. F. Hope-Stone, London Hospital, Depts. of Radiotherapy and Oncology, White Chapel, London E1 1BB/U.K.

G. Hortobágyi, see J. U. Gutterman

C. N. Hudson, Williasmon Laboratory, Medical College of St Bartholomew's Hospital, London EC1A 7BE/U.K.

P. Huguenin, see CMC de Bligny, F-91640 Briis sous Forges

M. Inbar, Department of Membrane Research, Weizmann Institute of Science, Rehovoth, Israel and Institut de Cancérologie et d'Immunogénétique (ICIG), Hôpital Paul-Brousse, 14–16, Avenue Paul-Vaillant-Couturier F-94800 Villejuif

S. Ingimarson, see H. Strander

L. Israel, Centre Hospitalier Universitaire, Hôpital Franco-Musulman, F-93000 Bobigny

R. Jackson, see S. E. Salmon

A. Jacobs, Welsh National School of Medicine, Heath Park, Cardiff, CF4 4XN/U.K.

E. M. Jacobs, see F. M. Muggia

C. Jacquillat, Hôpital Saint-Louis, 2, Place du Docteur-A. Fournier, F-75475 Paris-Cedex 10

C. Jasmin, EORTC Working Party Group, Institut de Cancérologie et d'Immunogénétique (ICIG), Hôpital Paul-Brousse, 14–16, Avenue Paul-Vaillant-Couturier, F-94800 Villejuif

J. A. Jefferies, see J. H. Edmonson

L. M. Jerry, see A. H. G. Paterson

R. Johnson, see S. E. Salmon

S. E. Jones, see S. E. Salmon

E. O. Jorgensen, see J. H. Edmonson

A. Jubert, St. Mary's Hospital, Grand Rapids, MI/USA

K. Karrer, Institut für Krebsforschung der Universität Wien, Borschkegasse 8A, A-Vienna

S. D. Kaufman, Harvard Medical School, Massachussets General Hospital, Cox Building, 100 Blossom Street, Boston 02115/USA

S. Kellar, see M. F. McKneally

J. A. Kellen, see J. W. Meakin

N. Kiger, see G. Mathé, (1)

D. J. Klaasen, see T. H. M. Stewart

F. Körner, see M. Hartmann

L. K. Kvols, see J. H. Edmonson

A. Lachand, Service d'Urologie, Hôpital Henri-Mondor, F-94000 Creteil

F. Lacour, Laboratoire d'Immunologie, Institut Gustave-Roussy, 16bis, Avenue Paul-Vaillant-Couturier, F-94800 Villejuif

J. Lacour, Service de Chirurgie, Institut Gustave-Roussy, 16 [bis], Avenue Paul-Vaillant-Couturier, F-94800 Villejuif

L. Lajtha, Christie Hospital and Holt Radium Institute, Paterson Laboratories, Manchester M20 9BX/U.K.

J. O. Lawton, see G. R. Giles

J. Lemerle, Départment de Pédiatrie, Institut Gustave-Roussy, 16bis, Avenue Paul-Vaillant-Couturier, F-94800 Villejuif

B. Le Mevel, Centre René Gauducheau, Quai Moncousu, F-44035 Nantes

D. Liegey-Bagarry, CRACM, Hôpital Sainte-Marguerite, F-13273 Marseille-Cedex

C. Lininger, see M. F. McKneally

E. Lopez-Cardozo, Free University, Amsterdam, The Netherlands

A. Louwagie, University of Leuven, B-3000 Leuven

D. Machin, see J. C. Goffin

D. Machover, see G. Mathé (1)

E. Mahon-Merlin, see F. Lacour

M. A. Malahy, see J. U. Gutterman

G. D. Malkasian, see J. H. Edmonson

A. Malkin, see J. W. Meakin

D. G. Malkin, see J. W. Meakin

C. Mangioni, Clinica Ostetrica Ginecologica, University of Milan, Italy

J. Maral, see C. Jacquillat

E. Margulis, see J. M. Zucker

B. Mason, see E. Stephens

G. Mathé, Institut de Cancérologie et d'Immunogénétique (ICIG), Hôpital Paul-Brousse (1), Service d'Hématologie de l'Institut Gustave-Roussy (2), 14–16, Avenue Paul-Vaillant-Couturier, F-94800 Villejuif

C. Mauer, see M. F. McKneally

R. Maurus, Hôpital Saint-Pierre, 320, Rue Haute, B-1000 Brussels

G. M. Mavligit, see J. U. Gutterman

M. Mayer, see E. Pommatau

A. Mazabraud, Fondation Curie, 26, Rue d'Ulm, F-75005 Paris

C. M. McBride, see J. U. Gutterman

M. F. McKneally, Division of Cardio-Thoracic Surgery, The Albany Medical College, Albany, NY 12208/USA

T. A. McPherson, see A. H. G. Paterson

J. W. Meakin, Ontario Cancer Institute and Sunnybrooke Medical Center, University of Toronto, 500 Sherbourne Street, Toronto, Ontario M4X 1K9/Canada

R. Metz, Centre Alexis Vautrin, F-54000 Nancy

G. Meyer, Institut Paolo-Calmettes, 232, Boulevard Sainte-Marguerite, F-13000 Marseille

A. M. Michelson, see F. Lacour

E. Mihich, Grace Cancer Drug Center, Roswell Park Memorial Institute, New York State Department of Health, Buffalo, NY 14263/USA

R. Miller, see S. E. Salmon

J. L. Misset, see G. Mathé (2)

P. Molteni, see C. Mangioni

S. Monfardini, Istituto Nazionale per lo Studio e la Cura dei Tumori, Via Venezian 1, I-2033 Milan

T. E. Moon, see S. E. Salmon

L. Morasca, Istituto Mario Negri, Via Eritrea, I-2033 Milan

G. Morello, Istituto Neurologico "C. Besta", I-2033 Milan

P. Morin, CMC de Bligny, F-91640 Briis sous Forges

K. Moser, see U. Ganzinger

S. E. M. Moss, see T. B. Grage

C. D. Mount, see X. Bertagna

F. M Muggia, Cancer Therapy Evaluation Program, Division of Cancer Treatment, National Cancer Institute, Bethesda, MD 20014/USA

J. H. Mulder, see L. M. van Putten

R. E. Myers, see J. W. Meakin

M. Namer, Centre Antoine-Lacassagne, 36, Avenue de la Voie Romaine, F-06000 Nice

W. E. Nicholson, see X. Bertagna

A. Nicolin, Institute of Pharmacology School of Medicine, Via Vanvitelli 32, I-2033 Milan

U. Nilsonne, see H. Strander

H. F. Oettgen, Memorial Sloan Kettering Institute Cancer Center, New York, NY 10021/USA

L. Olsson, Rigshospitalet, State University Hospital, 9 Blegdamsveg, DK-2100 Copenhagen

S. Orbach-Arbouys, see G. Mathé (1)

D. N. Orth, see X. Bertagna

J. Otten, see R. Maurus

T. Palangie, see P. Pouillart

Z. Palevic, see E. Mihich

A. H. G. Paterson, Department of Medicine, Cross Cancer Institute Edmonton, Alberta, Canada

C. Patte, see J. Lemerle

M. De Pauw, see C. Schulman

M. Pavone-Macaluso, Institute of Urology, University Polyclinic Hospital, Palermo, Italy

H. H. Peter, Medizinische Hochschule, D-3000 Hanover

O. S. Pettengill, see X. Bertagna

H. M. Pinedo, Oncology Unit, Department of Internal Medicine, University Hospital, Academish Ziekenhuis, Utrecht, The Netherlands

C. M. Pinsky, Memorial Sloan Kettering Cancer Center, New York, NY 10021/USA

R. Plagne, Centre Jean Perrin, Place Henri-Dunant, F-63000 Clermont-Ferrand

M. Poisson, Clinique Neurologique, Hôpital de la Salpétrière, 83, Boulevard de l'Hôpital, F-75013 Paris

E. Pommatau, Centre Léon Bérard, 28, Rue Laennec, F-69373 Lyon-Cedex 2

P. Pouillart, Service de Médecine Oncologique, Fondation Curie, 26, Rue d'Ulm, F-75005 Paris

T. A. Poulton, see C. N. Hudson

H. Pujol, Département de Chirurgie, Centre Paul Lamarque, Hôpital Saint-Eloi, F-34000 Montpellier

A. Puissant, see C. Jacquillat

G. A. Quash, Unité de Virologie Fondamentale et Appliquée, 1, Place Joseph Renaut F-69371 Lyon-Cedex 2

S. Raman, see T. H. M. Stewart

E. F. Rapp, see T. H. M. Stewart

A. Rey, see J. L. Amiel

P. Ribaud, see G. Mathé (1)

B. Richards, Department of Urology, York District Hospital, Wiggington Road, York Y03 7HE/U.K.

C. Rimbaud, see D. Buffe

J. P. Ripoll, Laboratoire de Biochimie, Hôpital Cardiovasculaire et Pneumologique, 59 Boulevard Pinel, F-69008 Lyon

R. A. Robins, see R. W. Baldwin

M. Robinson, Castleford Normanton and District Hospital, Castleford/U.K.

A. M. Roch, see G. A. Quash

S. A. Rosenberg, Surgery Branch, Radiation Oncology and Medical Oncology Branch, National Cancer Institute, Bethesda, MD 20014/USA

C. Rosenfeld, see G. Mathé (1)

R. Roy-Camille, Hôpital de la Pitié, 83, Boulevard de l'Hôpital F-75013 Paris

J. de Ruiter, see L. M. van Putten

Y. Rustum, see E. Mihich

H. J. Sachs, see T. H. M. Stewart

S. Saez, Laboratoire de Biologie Médicale, Centre Léon Bérard, 28, Rue Laennec, F-69373 Lyon-Cedex 2

M. J. Saffrey, see C. N. Hudson

R. Sagebiel, University of California School of Medicine, San Francisco 94143/USA

S. E. Salmon, Section of Hematology and Oncology, Arizona Health Sciences Center, 1501 N. Campbell Avenue, Tucson AZ 85724/USA

H. Sancho-Garnier, Département des Statistiques, Institut Gustave-Roussy, 16 bis, Avenue Paul-Vaillant-Couturier, F 94800 – Villejuif

H. Sauer, see W. Wilmans

C. Schaake, see E. Engelsman

A. Schalorn, Institut für Hämatologie, Gesellschaft für Strahlen- und Umweltforschung, Landwehrstraße 61, D-8000 Munich 2

Ph. S. Schein, see P. V. Wooley

M. Schneider, Centre Antoine-Lacassagne, 36, Avenue de la Voie Romaine, F-06000 Nice

C. Schulman, Service Universitaire, Hôpital Universitaire Brugmann, B-1020 Brussels

J. I. Schulz, see G. Mathé (1)

G. Schwaab, see J. L. Amiel

B. Serrou, Département de Chimio-Immunologie, Centre Paul-Lamarque, Hôpital Saint-Eloi, F-34000 Montpellier

G. A. Sisson, see S. G. Taylor

V. Slioussartchouck, see G. Mathé (1)

P. H. Smith, St James Hospital, Leeds LS9 7TF/U.K.

T. L. Smith, see J. U. Gutterman

S. Söderberg, see H. Strander

C. L. Solero, Istituto Neurologico "C. Besta", I-2033 Milan

G. D. Sorenson, Department of Pathology, Dartmouth Medical School, Hanover, NH 03755/USA

A. Spira, see F. Lacour

J. Stam, Free University of Amsterdam, Amsterdam, The Netherlands

M. Staquet, see C. Schulman

E. J. W. Stephens, Clinical Oncology Unit, Auckland Hospital, Park Road, Auckland 1, New Zealand

T. H. M. Stewart, Cancer Center, University of Ottawa, Ottawa Canada

J. Stines, Centre Alexis-Vautrin, F-54000 Nancy

J. Stjernswärd, Institut Ludwig de Recherches sur le Cancer, CH-1066 Epalinges s/Lausanne

H. Strander, Radiumhummet, Karolinska Hospital, S-104 01 Stockholm 60

M. Stromboni, see J. L. Amiel

E. W. Strong, Memorial Sloan Kettering Institute Cancer Center, New York, N.Y. 20007, USA

D. J. A. Sutherland, see J. W. Meakin

J. Swierenga, Saint Antonius Hospital, Utrecht, The Netherlands

R. Sylvester, EORTC Data Center, Institut Jules Bordet, 1, Rue Heger-Bordet, B-1020 Brussels

H. Szprirglas, Service de Stomatologie, CHU Pitié-Salpétrière, 47, Boulevard de l'Hôpital, F-75634 Paris-Cedex

T. Taguchi, Department of Oncology and Surgery, Institut for Microbial Diseases, Osaka Unit, Osaka, Japan

K. Tanaka, see X. Bertagna

Ch. K. Tashima, see J. U. Gutterman

S. G. Taylor, Section of Medical Oncology, Northwestern University Medical School, 303 E. Chicago Avenue, Chicago, Il 60611/USA

D. E. H. Tee, Department of Immunology, King's College Hospital, Denmark Hill, London S.E. 5/U.K.

M. F. Fournade, see J. Lemerle

A. Trifaud, Hôpital de la Conception, F-13000 Marseille

M. Tubiana, Département de Radiothérapie, Institut Gustave-Roussy, 16 bis, Avenue Paul-Vaillant-Couturier, F-94800 Villejuif

A. Vaghi, see G. Bonadonna

P. Valagussa, see G. Bonadonna

C. Vandenbrouck, Service d'ORL, Institut Gustave-Roussy, 16 bis, Avenue Paul-Vaillant-Couturier, F-94800 Villejuif

E. van Der Schueren, Department of Radiotherapy, Wilhelmina Gasthuis Eerste Helmerstraat 104, Amsterdam, The Netherlands

C. J. H. van de Velde, see L. M. van Putten

L. M. van Putten, Radiobiological Institute TNO, 151 Lange Kleiweg, Rijswijk, The Netherlands

F. de Vassal, see G. Mathé (1 and 2)

R. W. Veldhuizen, Free University, Amsterdam, The Netherlands

U. Veronesi, WHO Collaborating Centres for Evaluation of Methods of Diagnosis and Treatment of Melanoma, Istituto Nazionale dei Tumori, Via Venezian 1, I-2033 Milan

P. A. Voute, Emma Kinderziekenhuis, Amsterdam, The Netherlands

H. J. Wanebo, Department of Surgery, Unversity of Virginia Medical Center, Charlottesville, VA 22908/USA

C. Wastell, Westminster Hospital, London/U.K.

H. J. Webb, see J. H. Edmonson

A. Wendt, see S. E. Salmon

T. Wheeler, Addensbrooke's Hospital Cambridge, Cambridge/U.K.

P. Wibaut, see J. L. Amiel

D. Williams, see A. H. G. Paterson

W. Wilmans, Medizinische Klinik III, Klinikum Großhadern, Ludwig-Maximilians Universität München, Marchininistraße 15, D-8000 Munich 70

J. P. Wolff, Service de Gynécologie, Institut Gustave-Roussy, 16 bis, Avenue Paul-Vaillant-Couturier, F-94800 Villejuif

H. F. Wood, see E. Stephens

W. C. Wood, see S. D. Kaufman

P. V. Wooley, Department of Medicine, Division of Medical Oncology and Vincent I. Lombardi Cancer Research Center, Georgetown University Medical Center, Washington, DC 20007/USA

J. M. Zucker, Section Médicale, Fondation Curie, 26, Rue d'Ulm, F-75005 Paris

Introduction

P. Denoix and G. Mathé

Approximately 70% of cancer patients relapse after surgery before the 5th year and, in most cases, for example in breast carcinoma, they relapse still later up to the 20th year. For some considerable time, the strategy of cancer treatment has been limited to the sophistication of surgery-radiotherapy combinations that maximally decreased the incidence of local and regional relapses in sites that were within their reach.

Today, the practice of clinical oncology is unthinkable without the active participation of the medical oncologist. He is the "third man" of the clinical oncology team, and he has recently focused attention on the fact that most relapses arise from distant metastases due to the proliferation of cells seeded there after having left the primary tumor site at the time of operation and, hence, are inaccessible to any form of local and/or regional treatment. On this evidence, medical oncologists have proposed the application of medical treatments for disseminated minimal residual disease (MRD). They have two available means: chemotherapy and immunotherapy. Medical oncologists in general can be divided into three groups: chemotherapists, immunotherapists, and chemoimmunotherapists.

The pure chemotherapists, who had already cured some malignant neoplasias such as Hodgkin's disease, acute lymphoid leukemia, placental choriocarcinoma, and Wilms' tumor, thought they might have the means of attacking the residual disease of common cancers. Their preliminary results on osteosarcomas and breast cancer, which were spectacular, led us to believe that they had, indeed, the right drugs and only had to find the right methods of applying them. However, after a longer follow-up, we became disappointed since the benefit only remained significant for premenopausal breast carcinoma patients and decreased noticeably in osteosarcomas.

This evolution in the curves for osteosarcoma and postmenopausal breast carcinoma patients, demonstrating an early significant benefit that with time noticeably diminishes, evokes the notion that justifies research on immunotherapy, that chemotherapy does not kill "the last cell." As immunotherapy may kill the last cell on condition that the total number of neoplastic cells is small enough, immunotherapists first conducted trials of immunotherapy of postsurgical minimal residual disease in the case of neoplasias where chemotherapy has always, or in general, been unsuccessful. They obtained significant results, especially in carcinoma of the bronchus, melanoma, head and neck tumors, gastric carcinoma, and carcinoma of the cervix. They have conducted even more courageous trials cases of minimal residual disease of some cancers for which chemotherapy was claimed to be so successful, i.e., in breast carcinoma and osteosarcoma, and they also achieved beneficial results.

These two latter trials that immunotherapists dared to conduct on tumors, the problem of which appeared to have been improved by chemotherapy, are the most interesting. The comparison of the curves of the disease-free intervals generally shows a large initial difference between the chemotherapy branch and the control branch, while later on the difference is attenuated or the curves even converge. On the contrary, the curve of the immunotherapy branch is initially very close or identical to the curve of the controls but, subsequently, these two curves diverge.

This preliminary observation, which can be made on the overall data presented at this meeting, fits very well with the fact that chemotherapy obeys first-order kinetics and works even if there are many neoplastic cells left, but "does not kill the last cell," while immunotherapy may kill the entire population of neoplastic cells, but only if the total number is very small.

This observation is a complementary argument for conducting more trials where chemotherapy and immunotherapy are combined. Encouraging results have already been obtained with such combinations, not only in leukemia, but also in some solid tumors such as bronchial carcinoma, melanoma, and ovarian tumors.

Therefore, precisely as surgeons and radiotherapists have to cooperate on local and regional treatments, chemotherapists and immunotherapists, from now on, will also have to work together on the systemic treatment of the minimal residual disease. They have to cooperate not only to combine their means and to study the effects of chemotherapy on immunity and that of immunotherapy on pharmacology of oncostatics, but also to learn how to use the means that may work both as oncostatics and immunomodulators, such as interferon and the tumor necrosis factor.

Above all, there should not be two separate cooperative efforts: one of the "regionalists," i.e., surgeons and radiotherapists on the one hand, and one of the "systemists," i.e., chemotherapists and immunotherapists on the other. There should only be one cooperative effort: that of the four specialists, as postsurgical radiotherapy should not be applied systematically where it is not predicted as being useful or it may delay the systemic treatment predicted as being beneficial.

Similarly, chemotherapists should not systematically administer large doses of cytostatics to all cancer patients without knowing in detail all the characteristics of a particular disease and its prognosis, with the respective indication for chemotherapy, immunotherapy, combination chemo-immunotherapy, or abstention from any of them. Adjuvant medical therapy indications should not be systematic but established by the prognosis based on these characteristics. They are most often obtained by microscopic typing and by local topographic investigation of surgery that, when applied alone, cures a noticeable proportion of localized cancers. The surgeon may, in some cases, desire that a complementary treatment be given by radiotherapists to some area(s) where his operation does not give the guarantee of local cure; it is also the surgeon who gives data on the indication for adjuvant chemotherapy and/or immunotherapy. The most difficult problem that has to be discussed in some cases is the best moment for applying radiotherapy, and this can only be answered by trials involving cooperation of the four specialists of cancer treatment.

I. Incidence, Kinetics and Markers of Post-Surgical Minimal Residual Disease

Kinetics of Minimal Residual Disease

S. E. Salmon

Introduction

The development of a rational approach to adjuvant chemotherapy of cancer depends upon at least four factors:

1. Recognition that micrometastases are frequently disseminated and established prior to the time of surgery for a primary cancer;
2. Measurement (e.g., with biomarkers) or reliable estimates of the number of residual (and occult) clonogenic tumor cells remaining after surgery;
3. Knowledge of the kinetics behavior and drug sensitivity of small numbers of clonogenic cells;
4. Availability of effective anticancer drugs, particularly those that have a cell-cycle, nonspecific mode of action that will be lethal to quiescent cells as well as those undergoing proliferation.

In this analysis I will rely heavily on quantitative extrapolations relating to tumor kinetics and drug effects and select kinetic parameters characteristic of tumors that might be difficult to eradicate. This approach permits prediction of drug schedules and intensity of treatment that are likely necessary to eradicate the residual clonogenic tumor cell population. The Arizona Breast Cancer Adjuvant Program (results discussed elsewhere in this text) will be used to exemplify application of some of these principles.

Residual Tumor Burden and Tumor Mass Kinetics

For the present discussion, I consider adjuvant chemotherapy to be limited to the setting wherein less than 10^4 tumor cells remain after surgery. Once extremely sensitive and specific assays for tumor markers that detect 10^1–10^4 cells in the body are available, the problem of measuring the residual tumor burden will be enormously simplified. Unfortunately, none of the biomarkers currently available have this degree of sensitivity. However, while it is presently not possible to measure this small tumor burden directly, for certain common tumors it is possible to back-extrapolate from data relating to the time to relapse and estimate the residual burden of micrometastases after surgery. Such calculations require some knowledge of the cell-cycle time and growth kinetics of the particular cancer.
This approach to kinetic analysis has been used effectively by Skipper and Schabel [13]. One important aspect of their analysis was the recognition that the characteristic relapse or relapse-free survival curve for patients with any given type of cancer provided valuable insights about the residual tumor burden after primary surgery or radiotherapy. They assumed that both the time to recurrence and death were related to the number of tumor cells surviving primary surgery and/or irradiation. A typical curve of cancer recurrences after primary local treatment manifests an initially constant rate of recurrence for 1–3 years after

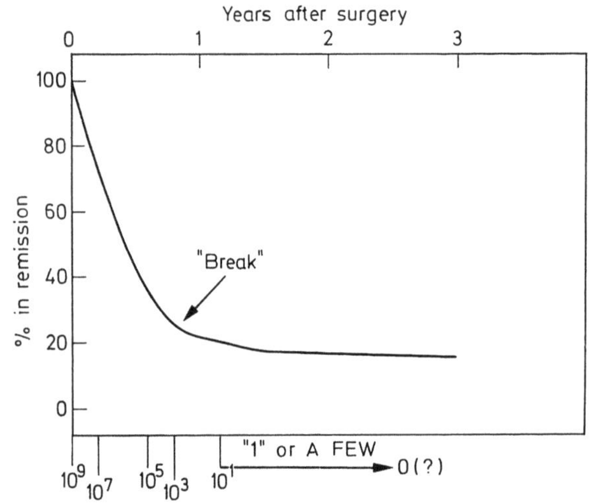

Fig. 1. Example of a "break" in freedom from relapse curve and its postulated relationship to tumor burden after surgery. For this hypothetic example, the median tumor doubling time was assumed to be 40 days. The residual tumor burden after surgery is depicted on the abscissa. In this example, patients relapsing beyond 1 year after surgery are estimated to have ten or fewer viable tumor cells remaining in the body immediately after surgery (reproduced with modification with permission of the authors) [13]

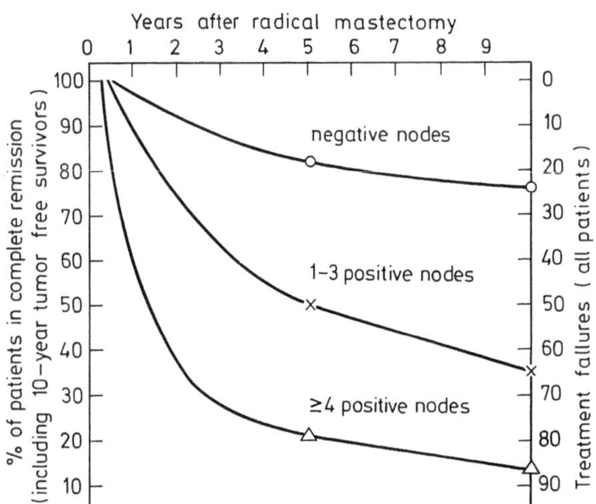

Fig. 2. The presumed relationship between lymph node status, prognosis, and residual tumor burden after surgery for women with stage I or II primary breast cancer who have undergone radical mastectomy. The average numbers of residual tumor cells at varying times after surgery can be estimated from this graph in relation to the degree of initial lymph node involvement (reproduced with modification with permission of the authors) [13]

primary therapy, followed by a decreasing rate of recurrence, and then a relatively flat component thereafter, reflecting the prolonged survival of the cohort of patients who were likely cured by the primary treatment (Fig. 1). SKIPPER and SCHABEL [13] identified the change in slope just prior to the flat component as the "break" in the survival curve, and postulated that it reflected the time for a minimal tumor burden (less than 10^1 tumor cells) to repopulate and present as metastatic disease.

Such curves were then related to tumor staging, and the relapse curve viewed as a titration of residual tumor burden after breast cancer surgery (Fig. 2). Additionally, it was proposed that if "just a few" tumor cells remain (e.g., one to three cells), the time to relapse may be exceptionally long because those few cells might not have typical growth characteristics, whereas if ten or more cells remained, the chance of a cell remaining with growth characteristics typical for the original tumor would be rather high. They went on to assume that the doubling time was relatively constant from 10^1–10^6 cells and calculated "median doubling times" (MDTs) for the repopulation phase so that they could then make predictions about the intensity of adjuvant chemotherapy that would be required.

While such calculations of MDTs are reasonable, they are estimated to be 40–60 days and are therefore considerably longer than the tumor generation time as measured with tritiated thymidine or the in vitro doubling time for tumor cells in agar cultures initiated at low dilutions. In these latter circumstances, the tumor doubling times are closer to 2–5 days. The biochemical explanation for increasing doubling time with increasing cell mass is uncertain and may be related to feedback regulatory factors. Available evidence suggests that the level of regulation is on the fraction of tumor stem cells that are capable of entering the proliferative cycle. For purposes of illustration of rational design of adjuvant chemotherapy programs, I have used computer analysis and modeled a tumor with Gompertzian kinetics, selecting an initial doubling time (one cell to two) of 2.34 days (about 56 h). The tumor growth curve is shown in Fig. 3, while Table 1 shows the calculated doubling times at various cell burdens.

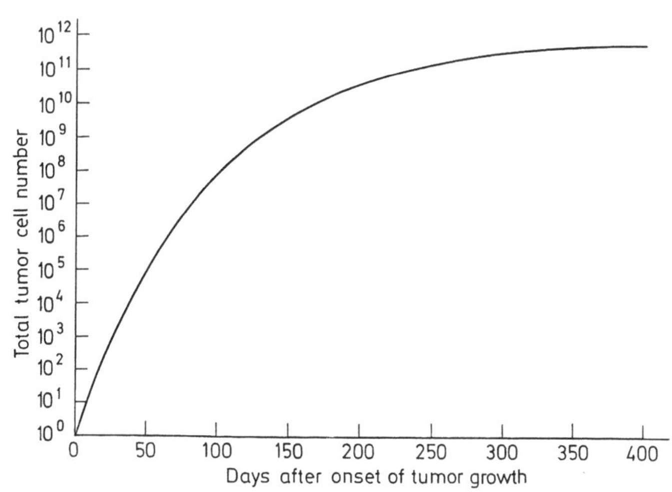

Fig. 3. A Gompertzian growth curve for a model of tumor mass behavior of human breast cancer. The initial doubling time (one cell to two) is set at 2.34 days (about 56 h). In this instance the term α in the Gompertz equation is set at 0.011 (see reference 14). Doubling times in relation to the log of tumor cell number are summarized in Table 1. The effects of chemotherapy after surgery on this growth curve are depicted in Fig. 5

Table 1. Total tumor burden and doubling times for the Gompertzian tumor growth curve for breast cancer depicted in Fig. 3

Log Tumor cell number		Doubling time
1×10^0	2×10^0	2.34 days
1×10^3	2×10^3	3.15 days
1×10^6	2×10^9	10.2 days
1×10^9	2×10^9	10.2 days
1×10^{11}	2×10^{11}	40.1 days

This same "model tumor" will be used subsequently for designing a treatment schedule for adjuvant breast cancer treatment.

Tumor Stem Cells: Measurements of Kinetics and Drug Sensitivity

The most important cells in a cancer are the colony-forming tumor stem cells, as they comprise the clonogenic self-renewal system required to maintain and propogate a cancer. Additionally, tumor stem cells are the seeds of metastasis, as they have the capability of migration and can initiate secondary colonies at distant sites. Viewed in that context, rational design of adjuvant chemotherapy could be simplifed by direct study of the kinetics and drug sensitivity of tumor stem cells present in primary cancers. Transplantable animal tumors or long passage in vitro tumor cell lines may not accurately reflect the proliferative behavior of the small compartment of tumor stem cells of an individual patient's primary cancer or its micrometastases. I take this view because the established tumor cell systems are of limited diversity in comparison to the clinical situations that the clinician sees with cancers that differ in histopathology, proliferative behavior, and susceptibility to anticancer drugs. To overcome this problem, studies of human tumor growth from biopsy samples have recently been undertaken in immunodeficient mice [11] and in vitro [3].

Several years ago, Anne Hamburger and I reported an in vitro soft agar colony-forming system that supports the growth of a variety of human tumors from patient biopsy samples [2, 3]. In this system, tumor cells are plated in relatively small numbers (5×10^5 cells) in semisolid agar along with conditioned medium. A small proportion of the tumor cells (0.01%–1.0%) from colonies of > 30 cells in 1–3 weeks. While some might argue that the cloning efficiencies that we have observed are too low and due to culture deficiencies, it is my belief that they may approximate the clinical situation. Similar low cloning efficiencies have been observed with soft agar culture of normal bone marrow progenitors both in vitro and in vivo. Additionally, many human tumors appear to undergo gradual evolution. As discussed above, the selective processes associated with serial passage and subculture of in vitro cell lines or transplantation in vivo would clearly favor enrichment of the clonogenic cells, and it is not surprising that higher plating efficiencies can be obtained with passaged tumor cells and that they can rapidly kill a host animal.

A summary of tumor types that we have successfully cloned directly from biopsy samples is summarized in Table 2. Evidence that the cultured cells are of malignant origin has been obtained with special stains, immune markers, and cytogenetics. A typical melanoma colony is shown in Fig. 4. We have yet to have significant success with breast cancer; however, a number of tumors appear to be quite amenable to clinical research on tumor cloning. For

Table 2. Human tumors types that have been directly cloned from biopsy samples[a]

Tumor type	Required incubation time
Myeloma	14 – 21 days
Non-Hodgkin's lymphoma	10 – 14 days
Melanoma	10 – 14 days
Neuroblastoma	10 days
Adenocarcinoma of ovary	7 – 10 days
Adenocarcinoma of endometrium	7 – 10 days
Adenocarcinoma of colon	7 – 10 days
Undifferentiated carcinoma (head and neck)	10 – 14 days
Small cell carcinoma of lung	10 – 14 days

[a] Data from references 2, 3, and 4 and subsequent unpublished experiments in our laboratory.

certain tumors (e.g., lymphomas), a different conditioned medium appears to be superior to the one we usually utilize [5].

For ovarian carcinoma, colonies of more than 30 cells are regularly present in 10 days, suggesting a potential doubling time in the clonogenic compartment of 2 days or less. Tritiated thymidine and hydroxyurea suicide experiments using a 1-h exposure to one of these S phase lethal agents have indicated that for most patients over half of the colony-forming cells are in S phase at the time of biopsy. Assuming that the S phase comprises over half of the total cycle time, > 90% of the tumor stem cells are in cycle. However, for other patients less than 20% of the clonogenic cells are actively in cycle at the time of collection, as less than 10% of the colony-forming cells are inactivated with high doses of ^{3}H-thymidine of hydroxyurea [4]. These observations would suggest to me that major reliance on cycle-active or cycle-phase-active drugs alone in adjuvant chemotherapy for breast cancer [7] and colorectal carcinoma [1] could yield far less than optimal results.

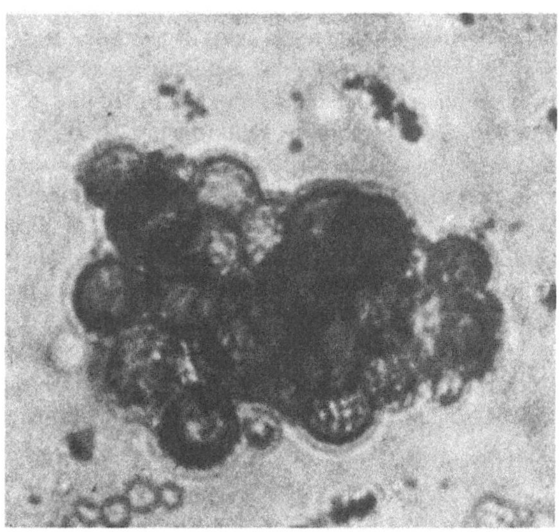

Fig. 4. A typical melanoma colony in soft agar culture 12 days after percutaneous biopsy and plating of a liver metastasis. Melanin granules can be seen in the cytoplasm of the cells. The needle biopsy sample was sufficient in size to also conduct a study of in vitro sensitivity to three anticancer drugs

Additionally, it appears that tumor kinetics as assessed with our clonogenic assays yield radically different results than those obtained with conventional ^{3}H-thymidine labeling autoradiography techniques. For example, in myeloma we commonly observe 1-h thymidine labeling indices in the range of 1.0% [2]. Nonetheless, when aliquots of the same samples are plated for myeloma colony formation, the same thymidine exposure can destroy anywhere from < 10% to > 75% of the clonogenic cells. These data imply that in some instances the clonogenic cells comprise up to 10% of the autoradiographically labeled cell population, whereas in other instances over 99% of the labeled cell population is unable to form colonies in our assay system. Conceivably, these DNA-synthesizing cells have differentiated sufficiently that they lack the ability to undergo an additional five to seven doublings. While technical problems related to viability have thus far limited our ability to make similar comparisons with cells marked for DNA content by flow microfluorimetry (FMF), I suspect that a similar lack of correlation with the clonogenic assay might be manifest. Conventional autoradiography and FMF have the limitation that the cells identified by these techniques may or may not be in the relevant clonogenic compartment. Therapeutic strategies based on the conventional kinetic techniques may therefore be incorrect.

Because of the problems with conventional techniques, we have focused on directly measuring the sensitivity of the freshly biopsied clonogenic tumor cells to anticancer drugs [8]. The quantitative assay technique that we developed involves a brief exposure (1 h) of cells in suspension to varying concentrations of a series of anticancer drugs that are biologically active in vitro. The cells are then washed and plated in standard fashion in agar culture and the reduction in the number of colony-forming cells determined with colony counts. A sensitivity index was devised based on measurement of the area under linear survival-concentration curves up to a boundary drug concentration defined in relation to pharmacologically achievable concentration time products (CXT) for the various agents. Patterns of differential sensitivity have been observed between patients with tumors of the same histology, and both drug-sensitive and drug-resistant cells have been observed within the population of tumor colony-forming cells from individual patients [8].

Our work on drug sensitivity in myeloma cases has shown over 20-fold range in melphalan sensitivity by human myeloma stem cells from different patients. This result should be viewed in relation to results in transplantable mouse myeloma, wherein differences of that magnitude in drug sensitivity in vitro were observed between different myeloma cell lines and correlated with in vivo sensitivity to the same drugs. Thus, each individual myeloma patient's stem cells may be as different from the next patient's as one transplantable myeloma tumor system is from another. Correlations between in vitro and in vivo sensitivity of myeloma and ovarian carcinoma to six common agents (melphalan, BCNU, adriamycin, vinblastine, methotrexate, and bleomycin) have recently been made [8]. These studies have suggested that the assay may prove useful in identifying drugs to which individual patients will manifest in vivo sensitivity or resistance. Additional studies will be required to determine the utility of this assay with other tumors and other drugs, as well as reproducibility in other centers. Nonetheless, a reasonable extrapolation from current techniques to adjuvant therapy would include routine tests of drug sensitivity of tumor stem cells from high-risk primary tumors resected at surgery. A feasible strategy would be to initiate a standardized adjuvant treatment for such patients and then alter it, if needed, based on in vitro patterns of sensitivity or resistance. This approach is of course similar to the current strategy for management of difficult bacterial infections.

Selection of Anticancer Drugs and Estimation of Tumor Cell Kill

Over 40 anticancer drugs are now available for clinical use, all of which have efficacy in one or more types of cancer. Selection of the appropriate agents for adjuvant therapy is not easy and thus far has required a good deal of empiricism. Certainly, it is logical to select agents capable of inducing remissions for advanced stages of the same type of cancer for which adjuvant therapy is contemplated. Other considerations also apply for adjuvant therapy. In general, we do not accept marked toxicity from adjuvant therapy programs because not all the patients treated assuredly have residual cancer. However, I believe that adjuvant programs should ideally be capable of reducing the size of the residual tumor stem cell population by 99%–99.9% per course. In part based on our tumor colony work, I think that major reliance should not be placed on cycle-specific drugs, as not all residual tumor stem cells are known to be in cycle or in the sensitive phase of the cycle at the time of drug administration. Cycle nonspecific agents generally manifest a dose-dependent "fractional cell kill" of the tumor stem cells exposed.

The magnitude of this fractional kill of stem cells (e.g., 90% or 99.9%) is grossly underestimated from tumor mass measurements in clinical trials in patients with advanced cancer. The conclusion that clinical tumor volume measurements grossly underestimate tumor stem cell kill is derived from several lines of evidence. Tumors are known to contain a number of components that contribute to volume but are not part of the tumor stem cell compartment. These include stromal elements such as blood vessels and connective tissue, differentiated tumor cells that have permanently lost capability of reentry into the proliferative compartment, and grossly necrotic tissue. Indeed, after administration of chemotherapy, there is a time delay of from days to months for physical dissolution of residual sterile tumor cells incapable of further division, as well as for resorption of the dead and dying elements in the tumor nodule and for involution of the stromal elements. Persistence of differentiated elements is perhaps best exemplifed in testicular cancers that may be effectively cured with combination chemotherapy but leave residual nonmalignant teratomas that may require subsequent surgical resection. Studies involving early transplantation of spontaneous animal tumors as well as studies of primary human tumors transplanted into nude mice and our recent studies of direct in vitro cloning suggest that only a small fraction of tumor cells (generally less than 1%) are capable of giving rise to tumor colonies. Extrapolating this to effects of chemotherapy, we might assume that a 10-g tumor nodule (10^{10} cells) contains 1% tumor stem cells (10^8 stem cells). In this situation, 3 log kill (99.9%) in the tumor stem cell compartment (which only contains 0.1 g) would be almost totally obscured initially by the remaining bulk of 9.9 g of tumor that would be subject to clinical measurement (lymph nodes, pulmonary metastases, etc.). In vivo studies such as those reported by Schabel [10] provide clear evidence that pharmacologically achievable concentrations of anticancer drugs cure animals with small tumor burdens and are sometimes capable of inducing multilog reductions in the number of tumor cells even in some tumors that may overtly appear to be resistant to treatment. However, drug sensitivity appears more important than tumor mass: choriocarcinoma in the female and ALL are often curable with chemotherapy even when they are present at an advanced stage. Use of combinations of effective drugs for adjuvant chemotherapy seems most reasonable and if the agents are selected carefully, additive or synergistic lethality to tumor cells may occur.

An argument can be made for inclusion of cycle-active agents in adjuvant chemotherapy if a significant number of residual tumor stem cells are triggered into cycle after ablation of the primary tumor. Autoradiographic evidence for such kinetic behavior has been gathered by

SIMPSON-HERREN and associates for a transplantable animal tumor system [12]. The emergence of drug-resistant mutants is likely a smaller problem quantitatively in the adjuvant setting than with advanced cancer, but even in the adjuvant setting the existence of a single drug-resistant tumor stem cell could cause relapse. Use of non-cross-resistant combinations of drugs with differing mechanisms of action should minimize the problem of repopulation by resistant mutants. Ideally, courses of treatment should be given sufficiently frequently to overcome apparent resistance that might be attributable to the kinetics of rapid tumor cell repopulation even by sensitive cells. Unfortunately, we do not have unequivocal data on tumor kinetics and the repopulation rates of specific human cancers over the range from one or a few viable tumor stem cells after surgery to a mass of 10^9–10^{10} cells, which likely would be manifest as one or a few overt metastases ("macrocolonies"). Hopefully, this type of information will be available in the future with the development of better biologic markers of tumor growth from very small numbers of cells. In the current analysis of the residual tumor stem cell problems, I assume that the initial doublings can be as rapid as they occur in vitro and that characteristic Gompertzian growth applies to the repopulation that adjuvant chemotherapy must eradicate. In our previous biologic marker studies of multiple myeloma, we have back-extrapolated from the clinical phase of tumor growth curves (from 10^{11} to 10^{12} cells) and predicted initial doubling times (10^0–2 to 10^0 cells) of 2–3 days. Our recent in vitro studies of myeloma colony doubling times now corroborate the earlier extrapolations from marker studies (Table 1).

While many of these comments are general, they were useful in designing our adjuvant breast cancer chemotherapy program at the University of Arizona, which I will review as an example of the application of our scientific rationale to a clinical trial. We chose to combine the cycle-nonspecific agents, adriamycin and cyclophosphamide, as in our own experience they were a very effective combination for use in advanced breast cancer and at several dosage levels induced a 60%–80% response rate, including about 15% complete responses. In experimental tumor systems, this combination appeared to cause a 2–3 log reduction in the number of tumor stem cells for certain neoplasms and was capable of curing some animals. These data also suggested that this drug combination might be synergistic or potentiating, i.e., with the combination exerting a greater effect than maximum dosage of either adriamycin or cyclophosphamide alone. Using the growth curve and kinetic constants described earlier (Fig. 3), we examined the effect of drug schedule, assuming that each course could induce a 99.7% cell kill. For these calculations we selected kinetics of an unfavorable tumor, with the view that the magnitude of the problem should not be underestimated.

As can be observed from the theoretical illustration in Fig. 5, starting with 10^3 residual cells after surgery, cure could be obtained with five courses of treatment administered every 3 weeks. In striking contrast, the micrometastases could not be eradicated if the treatment interval was increased to 4 weeks. In fact, with a 4-week schedule, gradual increase in the number of tumor stem cells will occur. Even if the kinetics of repopulation of breast cancer are not as vigorous as in the example we depicted, the effect of prolongation of the treatment intervals would nonetheless apply. NORTON and SIMON have performed a related analysis based on Gompertzian kinetics and proposed that treatment should be intensified before it is discontinued [6]. Inasmuch as we did not have any direct measurements of the lethality of the adriamycin-cyclophosphamide chemotherapy regimen on human breast cancer stem cells, it appeared reasonable to us to rigidly standardize the treatment schedule to every 3 weeks, as this length of time was necessary for adequate repopulation of normal hematopoietic progenitors. We are hopeful that in the future in vitro bioassay of human tumor colony-forming cells will permit direct measurement of drug sensitivity on biopsy samples of the primary tumor. In

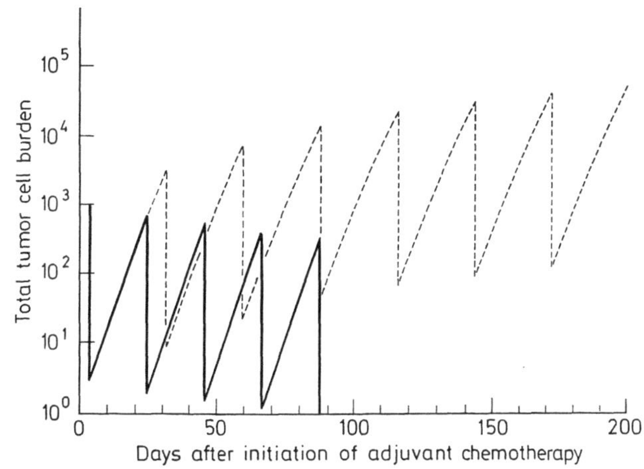

Fig. 5. Effect of treatment schedule (dose rate) on the ability to eradicate a residual burden of 10^3 tumor cells after surgery for breast cancer. The underlying tumor mass growth curve is identical to that depicted in Fig. 3. Each perpendicular line on the growth curves is meant to reflect a 99.7% reduction in tumor burden with each course of chemotherapy. For this very difficult tumor, treatment at 3-week intervals resulted in cellular cure within five cycles of treatment. In contrast, with a standardized treatment of this intensity delivered every 4 weeks, cure could not be accomplished irrespective of the number of cycles of treatment. This latter schedule would also provide longer opportunity for the emergence of a drug-resistant subclone

light of SKIPPER and SCHABEL'S analysis of the relationship of lymph node involvement to the number of residual tumor cells after surgery (Fig. 2), we chose to administer differing numbers of cycles of adjuvant chemotherapy based on lymph node (and primary tumor) status and risk of recurrence. Thus, patients with stage I breast cancer only receive three cycles of adjuvant chemotherapy (90 mg/m^2 of adriamycin), whereas patients with stage II disease receive eight cycles of treatment (240 mg/m^2 of adriamycin) and complete adjuvant therapy approximately 6 months after mastectomy. As will be discussed elsewhere in this text [9], the early results of this program are quite encouraging, but we will need additional years of follow-up to adequately assess the utility of this specific adjuvant program, particularly in the stage I cases.

Similar rationale can likely be applied to development of adjuvant programs for a variety of other forms of cancer. In some instances, systemic or regional chemotherapy might be more appropriately started preoperatively. However, in that setting, early surgery should be contemplated because a large tumor burden exposed to chemotherapy may set the stage for the undesired selection of drug-resistant mutant colonies that could persist after surgery.

Sanctuary Problem

Even with effective anticancer drugs of adequate potency, certain neoplasms appear particularly prone to "the sanctuary problem" due to seeding of tumor stem cells to specific sites. This problem was first observed in childhood acute lymphocytic leukemia (ALL) wherein central nervous system (CNS) relapse was a major site of recurrent disease in patients in peripheral remission. This effect clearly appears to be due to the blood-brain barrier and results from failure of adequate drug permeation to the meninges and brain substance. This problem has now been overcome in most ALL patients with intrathecal chemotherapy and whole brain radiotherapy administered prophylactically to eradicate a few occult stem cells. With the improvement in systemic therapy that is now observed in a variety of other neoplasms (e.g., oat cell carcinoma, diffuse histiocytic lymphoma, breast cancer), it has become apparent that the CNS sanctuary problem is important in these tumors as well and will need to be addressed for a variety of cancers with known propensity for CNS metastasis. The extent to which CNS therapy becomes a part of adjuvant chemotherapy programs will undoubtedly be dependent on the patterns of recurrence that are observed in patients who relapse on some of the current adjuvant chemotherapy trials. Sanctuaries such as the brain need not act only as a site of relapse. Conceivably, a site such as the CNS could serve as a reservoir for reseeding tumor stem cells to other systemic sites that offer more favorable growth conditions for tumor cells.

Acknowledgement

I wish to thank Drs. Frank Schabel and Howard Skipper for allowing me to reprint Fig. 2 and 3 and Drs. Stephen E. Jones, Anne Hamburger, Brian Durie, and David Alberts for their superb collaboration in various aspects of this work. The author's work was supported in part by USPHS grant CA 17094 and CA 21839 from the National Cancer Institute, Bethesda, Maryland 20014.

References

1. Grace, T. B., Metter, G. E., Cornell, G. N., et al.: The role of 5-fluorouracil as an adjuvant to the surgical treatment of large bowel cancer. In: Adjuvant therapy of cancer. Salmon, S., Jones, S. (eds.), pp. 259–264. Elsevier, North-Holland 1977
2. Hamburger, A., Salmon, S. E.: Primary bioassay for human myeloma stem cells. J. Clin. Invest. *60*, 846 (1977)
3. Hamburger, A., Salmon, S. E.: Primary bioassay of human tumor stem cells. Science. *197*, 461 (1977)
4. Hamburger, A. W., Salmon, S. E., Kim, M. B., et al.: Direct cloning of human ovarian carcinoma cells in agar. Cancer Res. *38*, 3438 (1978)
5. Jones, S. E., Hamburger, A. W., Salmon, S. E.: Development of a bioassay for human putative lymphoma stem cells. Blood (1979) (in press)
6. Norton, L., Simon, R.: Tumor size, sensitivity to therapy and design of treatment schedules. Cancer Treatment Rep. *61*, 1307 (1977)
7. Ramirez, G., Ansfield, F. J., et al.: Adjuvant chemotherapy-radiotherapy in breast carcinoma. In: Adjuvant therapy of cancer. Salmon, S., Jones, S. (eds.), pp. 165–170. Elsevier, North-Holland 1977
8. Salmon, S. E., Hamburger, A. W., et al.: Quantitation of differential sensitivity of human-tumor stem cells to anticancer drugs. New Engl. J. Med. *298*, 1321–1327 (1978)
9. Salmon, S. E., Wendt, A., Jones, S. E., et al.: Treatment of early breast cancer with adriamycin-cyclophosphamide with or without radiation therapy: Initial results of a brief and effective adjuvant program. In: Recent Results in Cancer Research, Vol. 68. Bonadonna, G., Mathé, G., Salmon, S. E. (eds.), pp. 98–104. Berlin, Heidelberg, New York: Springer 1979

10. Schabel, F. M. (Jr.): Experimental basis for adjuvant chemotherapy. In: Adjuvant therapy of cancer. Salmon, S., Jones, S. (eds.), pp. 3–15. Elsevier, North-Holland 1977
11. Shimosato, Y., et al.: Transplantation of human tumors in nude mice. J. Natl. Cancer Inst. *56,* 1251 (1976)
12. Simpson-Herren, L., Sanford, A., Holmquist, J.: Effects of surgery on the cell kinetics of residual tumor. Cancer Treat. Rep. *60,* 1749 (1976)
13. Skipper, H., Schabel, F. (Jr.): Quantitative and cytokinetics studies in experimental tumor systems. In: Cancer medicine, 2nd ed. Holland, J. F., Frei, E., III (eds.). Philadelphia: Lea and Febiger 1979 (in press)
14. Sullivan, P. W., Salmon, S. E.: Kinetics of growth and regression of IgG multiple myeloma. J. Clin. Invest. *51,* 1697 (1972)

Ectopic Production of ACTH, Lipotropin, and β-Endorphin by Human Cancer Cells. Structurally Related Tumor Markers

X. Y. Bertagna, W. E. Nicholson, K. Tanaka, C. D. Mount, G. D. Sorenson, O. S. Pettengill, and D. N. Orth

Introduction

Ectopic hormone secretion was first demonstrated by Meador et al. [8] in 1962 in patients with Cushing's syndrome due to ACTH production by nonpituitary tumors. Since this discovery almost all the known peptide hormones have now been reported to be ectopically produced by a variety of tumors (Table 1). This new concept has lead to major developments in endocrinology, particularly in the field of peptide hormone biosynthesis. On the other hand, it has stimulated the search for a new class of tumor markers (hormone markers) with potential usefulness in cancer detection, localization, and therapeutic evaluation.

Since by definition an ectopic hormone is produced by cells that do not *normally* secrete this hormone, it should be emphasized that certain criteria are necessary for diagnosis [16], among them:

1. decreased plasma hormone concentration after tumor removal;
2. no modification of plasma hormone concentration after removal of the gland *normally* secreting the hormone;
3. presence of an arteriovenous plasma hormone concentration gradient across the tumor bed;

Table 1. Reported ectopic hormones

Ectopic hormone	Site of tumor
ACTH	Lung, thymus, carcinoid, breast, pancreas, thyroid, liver, prostate, colon, adrenal
ADH	Lung, pancreas, duodenum, uterus
Calcitonin	Breast, lung, stomach
Enteroglucagon	Kidney
Erythropoietin	Uterus, cerebellar hemangioblastoma
FSH	Lung
GH	Lung, stomach
Glucagon	Bronchus, kidney
HCG and HCG α, β-subunits	Lung, liver, pancreas, stomach
Human placental lactogen	Lung
Insulin	Lung
LH	Lung, liver
Prolactin	Bronchus, kidney
PTH	Bronchus, kidney, ovary, endometrium, breast, cervix, vulva, esophagus
TSH	Bronchus, breast

Data taken mainly from Rees and Ratcliffe [16].

4. presence of high concentration of hormone in tumor tissue; and
5. in vitro secretion and synthesis of the hormone by the tumor cells in tissue culture.

Although an ideal ectopic hormone tumor marker (i.e., tumor specific, highly sensitive, present in all cases, reflecting the actual tumor mass and response to therapy) has not yet been found, a large body of evidence suggests that hormone blood measurement may prove useful for cancer detection and therapy, at least in certain circumstances. In this regard, hormones of placental origin, human chorionic gonadotropin (HCG) and its subunits and human placental lactogen (HPL), have been the most extensively studied in man [18] in different types of cancer. Their plasma concentrations may often reflect tumor status. However, dissociations have also been reported, particularly tumor growth without a corresponding increase in blood hormone concentration [18].

The potential use of immunoreactive ACTH as a tumor marker was described by AYVAZIAN et al. [1], who found increased plasma immunoreactive (IR) ACTH in a large percent of patients with lung cancer. Hormone concentration tended to be lower in treated patients. Together with the finding of GEWIRTZ and YALOW [3] that IR-ACTH was present in almost all lung tumor tissue extracts that they examined, these data suggested that the incidence of ectopic ACTH secretion might be much higher than had been estimated by LIDDLE et al. [6] and might, therefore, be of considerable interest in cancer detection.

Many observations suggest that ectopically produced hormones may have molecular forms different from those found in the normal tissue of origin. YALOW first reported the presence of "big ACTH" in tumor extracts and in plasma of patients with the ectopic ACTH syndrome [21]. Fragments of the (1-39) ACTH molecule also appear to be secreted by ectopic ACTH-producing tumors [13, 16].

Following the elegant studies by MAINS and EIPPER [7] and ROBERTS and HERBERT [17] on ACTH biosynthesis in the mouse pituitary tumor cell line AtT-20/D-16v, a new concept has evolved that guided our research on the exact nature of big ACTH in man (Fig. 1). These authors have demonstrated that the AtT-20 cells synthesize a high molecular weight glycopeptide precursor molecule that contains the sequence of both ACTH and β-lipotropin (or β-LPH). β-LPH has as its carboxy terminal sequence the endogenous opiate peptide, β-endorphin (β-END). The amino terminal sequence of β-LPH is γ-LPH. ACTH, β-LPH, and β-END, as well as intermediate fragments, appear to be cleaved from the common precursor molecule by selective proteolysis and subsequently secreted by the AtT-20 cell.

We wanted to investigate whether such a biosynthetic model might also exist in man. Our goal was to characterize further the exact nature of human big ACTH as well as other structurally related peptides that may be secreted concomitantly by ectopic ACTH-producing tumors. Hopefully, such studies would lead to the finding of new tumor markers. Thus, we examined the secretion products of human cancer cells derived from an oat cell carcinoma of the lung that had been established in continuous tissue culture. For this purpose, we used three radioimmunoassays (RIAs), for ACTH, hLPHs, and h-β-END. Plasma from a patient with the ectopic ACTH syndrome due to pancreatic carcinoma was also examined with the h-β-END RIA.

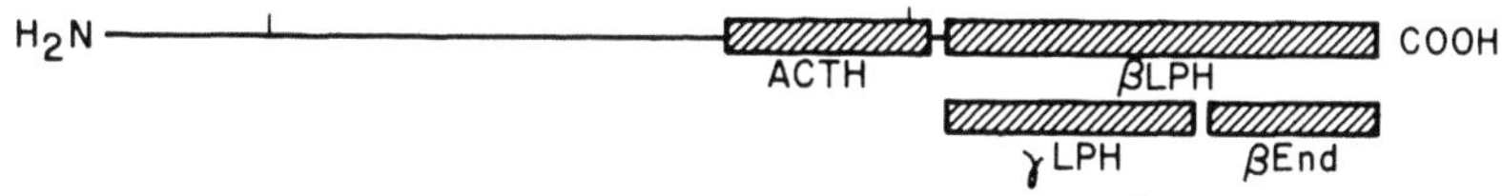

Fig. 1. Postulated common biosynthetic precursor for ACTH, β-LPH, γ-LPH, and β-END

Material and Methods

Human Cell Culture

The DMS-79 cell line originated from pleural fluid obtained from a patient with a diagnosis of small cell anaplastic carcinoma of the lung [PETTENGILL, SORENSON, MAURER, in preparation]. Cells were grown in stationary suspension in RPMI 1640 medium (Grand Island Biological Co., Grand Island, NY) with 20% fetal calf serum (Rehatuin®, Reheis Chemical Co. Kankakee, IL, heat inactivated at 56° for 30 min).

Radioimmunoassays

ACTH RIA

The ACTH RIA, using an anti-ACTH serum (S_1B_2) directed toward the 11–24 sequence of ACTH, was performed as previously described [13] except that separation of antibody-bound from free hormone was achieved by precipitation with a second antibody (Cappel Laboratories, Inc., Cochranville, PA).

Human β-END RIA

The h-β-END RIA, using an antiovine β-END serum (RB100-11/15) kindly provided by GUILLEMIN [4], was performed in an identical manner except that synthetic h-β-END (Bachem, Inc., Torrance, CA) was used both as tracer and standard. Both h-β-END and h-β-LPH react on an equimolar basis in this assay.

Human LPH RIA

The hLPH RIA procedure, using antiserum R-3 [14] and synthetic (37-58) hLPH ("human β-MSH", CIBA-GEIGY, Ltd., Basel Switzerland) as tracer and standard, was identical to that of ACTH RIA. Both β-LPH and γ-LPH are detected by this assay. On a molar basis their cross reactivities are 20% and 68%, respectively, as compared to the synthetic (37–58) hLPH standard.

Gel Filtration Chromatography

A 1.5 × 90 cm column was packed with Sephadex G-50 fine gel (Pharmacia), equilibrated, and developed in 0.05 M phosphate buffer pH 7.4 containing ACTH-free human plasma (10 ml/liter) and lysozyme (1 g/liter). Flow rate was 22 ml/h under 40 cm hydrostatic pressure; 2.2 ml fractions were collected and stored at −70° until assay. The following reagents were used to calibrate the column: bovine serum albumin (BSA) as a void volume marker; highly purified h-β-LPH and h-γ-LPH (kindly provided by LI and LOWRY, respectively); synthetic ACTH (CIBA-GEIGY), (37–58) hLPH, and h-β-END; and NaCl as a total volume marker.

Gel Filtration Chromatography Under Denaturing Conditions

A 1.5 × 90 cm column was packed with cross-linked agarose resin (Sepharose® CL-6B, Pharmacia), equilibrated, and developed at 4° with 6 *M* guanidine-HCl (GDN-HCl, Ultrapure, Schwarz-Mann, Orangeburg, NY), 0.1 *M* Na_2HPO_4, containing 200 mg BSA per liter, pH adjusted to 7.0 with 1 *M* NaOH. One milliliter of sample or calibration standard was applied and eluted by ascending flow (15 ml hydrostatic pressure) at a flow rate of 1.33 ml/cm²/h. The column was calibrated with: blue dextran 2000 (Pharmacia) as a void volume marker, reduced and carboxymethylated ovalbumin (Sigma Chemical Co., St. Louis, MO); reduced and carboxymethylated myoglobin (type II, whale skeletal muscle, Sigma); cytochrome C (type VI, horse heart, Sigma), highly purified h-β-LPH and h-γ-LPH; synthetic ACTH, ^{125}I-h-β-END and (37–58) hLPH; and dinitrophenyl (DNP) alanine (Sigma) as a total volume marker. Each sample or standard was incubated in the 6 *M* GDN-HCl buffer for 18 h at 4° prior to application; protein concentration was 3%. Each sample contained blue dextran 2000 and DNP alanine as internal markers.

Affinity Chromatography

Synthetic (1–24) ACTH was coupled to CNBr-Sepharose 4B gel (Pharmacia) and used to purify anti-ACTH antibody obtained in a rabbit immunized with (1–24) ACTH conjugated to BSA using glutaraldehyde [9]. Purified antibody was then reacted with CNBr-Sepharose 4B. A column was prepared with Sepharose-bound anti-(1-24) ACTH antibody. Specificity of the column was tested with freshly labeled peptides: ^{125}I-hACTH was completely adsorbed to the column and eluted only with 6 *M* GDN-HCl pH 1.5; in contrast, ^{125}I-h-β-LPH, ^{125}I-h-γ-LPH, and ^{125}I-h-β-END were almost totally excluded from the column.

Results

Radioimmunoassays

Serial dilutions of pooled medium in which DMS-79 cells had been cultured generated competitive binding curves parallel to those of the standard peptides in all three RIAs. Concentrations of IR ACTH, IR hLPH, and IR h-β-END in the medium were 10.5, 2.24, and 7.34 ng/ml, respectively.

Sephadex G-50 Gel Filtration Chromatography of DMS-79 Culture

Medium

Gel fractionation of culture medium on Sephadex G-50 revealed several different components that were responsible for the observed immunoreactivities of the medium in the three RIAs (Fig. 2). Starting with the materials that eluted first, there was:

1. a high molecular weight (HMW) component(s) that had ACTH; h-β-END and hLPH immunoreactivities;

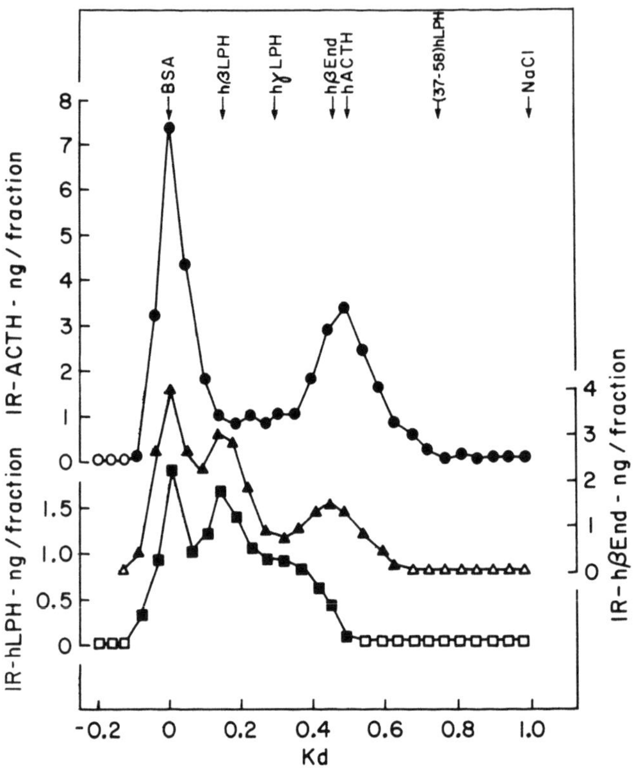

Fig. 2. Sephadex G-50 gel filtration chromatography of DMS-79 culture medium. Culture medium was diluted with an equal volume of glacial acetic acid, heated at 100° for 10 min, diluted with four volumes of distilled water, and lyophilized; the powder was stored at −70°. The equivalent of 10 ml original medium was reconstituted in 4 ml distilled water, aliquots were removed for hormone RIA, and the remaining 3.7 ml were applied to the 1.5 × 90 cm G-50 column and eluted. The 2.2 ml fractions collected were stored at −70° until assayed in the three different RIA systems. Recoveries of IR hACTH (●–●), IR h-β-END (▲–▲), and IR hLPH (■–■) were 82%, 76%, and 132%, respectively.

Elution volumes of BSA; purified h-β-LPH and h-γ-LPH, synthetic h-β-END, hACTH and (37–58) hLPH; and NaCl calibration standards are indicated. The abscissa represents the fractional elution volume (Kd) between the void volume and the total volume of the column. The open symbols in this and subsequent figures represent nondetectable immunoreactivity at the concentration plotted

2. a component that coeluted with h-β-LPH and had both h-β-END and hLPH immunoreactivities and appeared, therefore, to be a substance similar to h-β-LPH itself;
3. a shoulder of IR hLPH that coeluted with h-γ-LHP and thus appeared to be a substance similar to h-γ-LPH;
4. a peak of IR h-β-END that coeluted with synthetic h-β-END; and
5. a peak of IR ACTH that eluted in the same volume as synthetic hACTH. No IR-hLPH component that eluted in the position of synthetic.

(37-58) hLPH (an artifactual fragment of hLPH previously thought to represent "human β-MSH") was observed.

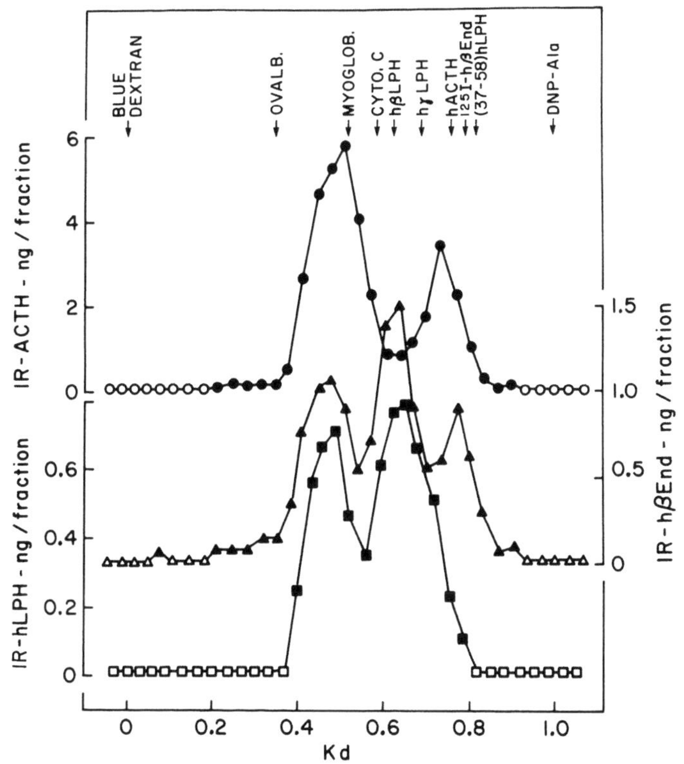

Fig. 3. Sepharose CL-6B chromatography of DMS-79 culture medium in 6 *M* GDN-HCl. Lyophilized medium (81.6 mg, equivalent to 36 mg protein) was dissolved in 1.2 ml 6 *M* GDN-HCl in 0.1 *M* phosphate buffer, pH 7.0, containing 2.0 mg blue dextran 2000 and 0.250 mg DNP alanine, and was incubated at 4° for 18 h. Four 50-μl aliquots were removed to determine their immunoreactive hormone content, and the remainder (1.0 ml) was applied to the column and eluted. Alternate fractions and the 50-μl aliquots were desalted and assayed in the three RIAs. Recovery of IR ACTH (●—●), IR h-β-END (▲—▲), and IR hLPH (■—■) were 87%, 98%, and 83%, respectively. The elution volumes of blue dextran 2000; ovalbumin; myoglobin; cytochrome-C; purified h-β-LPH and h-γ-LPH; synthetic hACTH, ^{125}I-h-β-END, and (37—58) hLPH; and DNP alanine calibration standards are indicated

Sepharose CL-6B/GDN-HCl Gel Filtration Chromatography of DMS-79

Culture Medium

The same immunoreactive components were observed under denaturing conditions (Fig. 3). The HMW material(s) with ACTH, hLPH, and h-β-END immunoreactivities eluted as a broad peak in the molecular weight range of about 15,000—40,000 daltons (Kd = 0.40—0.53). Substances similar to h-β-LPH, hACTH, and h-β-END were again observed, and probably an h-γ-LPH-like substance, although it was not clearly separated from the h-β-LPH-like component in this system.

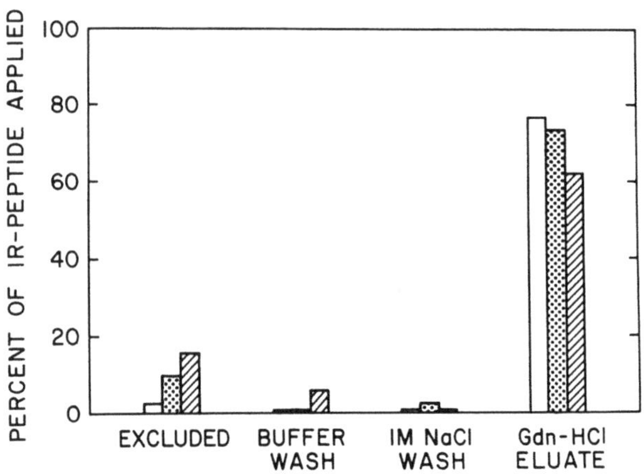

Fig. 4. Affinity chromatography of the high molecular weight IR ACTH/hLPH/h-β-END component from the CL-6B/GDN-HCl column. Even-numbered fractions between 0.40–0.53 Kd from the CL-6B/GDN-HCl column were desalted and pooled. Aliquots were removed for RIAs and the remainder was applied to the ACTH immune affinity column. The following four fractions were collected: the excluded sample, two washes and the fraction eluted with 6 *M* GDN-HCl, pH 1.5. The 1 *M* NaCl wash and GDN-HCl eluate were desalted on 1.1 × 26 cm Sephadex G-10 columns, and the IR hormone content of each fraction and that of the applied sample was determined in the same assay in each of three RIAs. Recoveries of IR hACTH (□), IR h-β-END (▩), and IR hLPH (▨) were 80%, 87%, and 86%, respectively. Recovery of freshly purified ^{125}I-hACTH, applied with the sample, was 80%

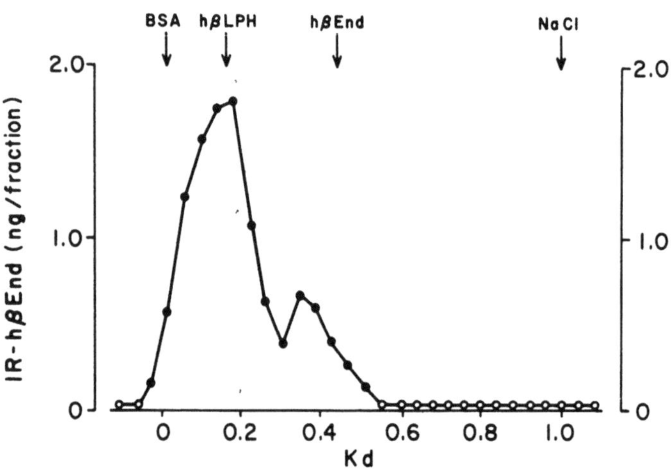

Fig. 5. Sephadex G-50 gel filtration chromatography of plasma from a patient with the ectopic ACTH syndrome. Lyophilized plasma 125 mg from a patient with the ectopic ACTH syndrome due to pancreatic carcinoma was reconstituted in column buffer and subjected to gel fractionation as in Fig. 1. Alternate collected fractions were assayed for IR h-β-END. Recovery of IR h-β-END was 95%

Immune Affinity Chromatography

When pooled fractions from the HMW region (Kd = 0.40—0.53) of the Sepharose CL-6B/GDN-HCl column (Fig. 3) were applied to the anti-ACTH affinity column, less than 17% of the IR ACTH, IR hLPH, or IR h-β-END were excluded, no more than 7% was recovered in the washes, and similar percentages of each (77%, 63%, and 74%, respectively) were eluted only with acidified 6 *M* GDN-HCl (Fig. 4).

Sephadex G-50 Gel Filtration Chromatography of Plasma from a Patient with the Ectopic ACTH Syndrome

Gel fractionation of the plasma from a patient with the ectopic ACTH syndrome revealed that at least two components were responsible for the observed β-END immunoreactivity (Fig. 5). A large component coeluting with h-β-LPH accounted for approximately 80% of total β-END immunoreactivity; a smaller component coeluting with h-β-END accounted for the other 20% of total immunoreactivity.

Discussion

There is already some evidence that human HMW ACTH may represent hormone precursor(s) analogous to the HMW ACTH synthesized by mouse AtT-20/D-16v pituitary tumor cells:

1. HMW ACTH components have been identified by gel filtration chromatography in human plasma and extracts of normal pituitary tissue and nonpituitary tumor tissues [5, 12];
2. HMW LPH, in addition to β-LPH and γ-LPH, has been identified by the same technique in similar specimens [2, 5, 19];
3. HMW ACTH can be converted to a biologically active molecule about the size of (1—39) ACTH by mild trypsin digestion [2];
4. HMW ACTH has been shown to be a glycopeptide on the basis of concanavallin A affinity chromatography [11];
5. ACTH, β-LPH, γ-LPH, β-END, and a HMW component with both ACTH and LPH immunoreactivity have been demonstrated in an extract of a pancreatic islet cell carcinoma [10].

However, there has been no human model system analogous to the AtT-20/D-16v cell line in which to examine the biosynthetic relationships of these peptide products.

We have studied the secretion products of human cancer cells derived from an oat cell carcinoma of the lung (DMS-79). Interestingly, although the patient from which the cells were obtained was not diagnosed as having hypercortisolism, the cultured cells were found to produce IR ACTH. Thus, this cell line appeared to provide a potential model in which to examine ectopic production of ACTH and structurally related peptides (β-LPH, γ-LPH, and β-END) in man.

Indeed, examination of the DMS-79 culture medium with three different RIAs revealed the presence of substances immunologically related to ACTH, LPHs and β-END. However, precise characterization of the materials responsible for the observed immunoreactivities required their physical separation. Molecular sieving demonstrated the presence of at least five different peptides: ACTH, β-LPH, γ-LPH and β-END. In addition, there was a HMW component(s) that had ACTH, LPH, and β-END immunoreactivity. The observation that all three immunoreactivities were still present in the HMW material(s) under denaturing conditions indicated that they might all be contained in the same molecule(s). Immune affinity chromatography demonstrated that the HMW material(s) with hLPH and h-β-END immunoreactivities also possessed an ACTH antigenic site. These data suggest that ectopic synthesis of ACTH and the related peptides, LPHs and β-END, in man may proceed in a manner similar to that proposed in mouse pituitary cells (Fig. 1).

Big ACTH [5, 13, 20], β-LPH, and γ-LPH [19] have been detected in the blood of patients with cancer. Thus far, there has been no report of circulating β-END in man. Our data show not only that β-END can be secreted ectopically by human cancer cells, but suggest that detectable concentrations of h-β-END or closely related peptides may circulate in the blood of patients with the ectopic ACTH syndrome. Depending upon the circulating half-life of these peptides in plasma, they may provide yet another useful marker for certain patients with cancer.

Acknowledgement

The authors thank Dr. Dr. Guillemin for the generous gift of antiovine β-END serum; Drs. C. H. Li and P. J. Lowry for providing us with highly purified h-β-LPH and h-γ-LPH, respectively; CIBA-GEIGY, Ltd., Basel, Switzerland for the supply of synthetic hACTH, (37-58) hLPH, and α-MSH; and Ms. Barbara Sherrell for her excellent technical assistance. This study was supported in part by National Cancer Institute Research Grants CA11685 and CA17710, NIH Research Grant AMO5318, USPHS General Research Support Grant RR03592, and a grant from the Hitchcock Foundation, Hanover, NH. X.Y.B. is an Eli Lilly International Research Fellow.

References

1. Ayvazian, L. F., Schneider, B., Gewirtz, G., Yalow, R. S.: Ectopic production of big ACTH in carcinoma of the lung. Its clinical usefulness as a biologic marker. Am. Rev. Resp. Dis. *111*, 279–287 (1975)
2. Gewirtz, G., Schneider, B., Krieger, D. T., Yalow, R. S.: Big ACTH: conversion to biologically active ACTH by trypsin. J. Clin. Endocrinol. Metab. *38*, 227–230 (1974)
3. Gewirtz, G., Yalow, R. S.: Ectopic ACTH production in carcinoma of the lung. J. Clin. Invest. *53*, 1022–1032 (1974)
4. Guillemin, R., Ling, N., Vargo, T.: Radioimmunoassays for α-Endorphin and β-Endorphin. Biochem. Biophys. Res. Commun. *77*, 361–366 (1977)
5. Himsworth, R. L., Bloomfield, G. A., Coombes, R. C., Ellison, M., Gilkes, J. J. H., Lowry, P. J., Setchell, K. D. R., Slavin, B., Rees, L. H.: "Big ACTH" and Calcitonin in an ectopic hormone secreting tumor of the liver. Clin. Endocrinol. *7*, 45–62 (1977)
6. Liddle, G. W., Nicholson, W. E., Island, D. P., Orth, D. N., Abe, K., Lowder, S. C.: Clinical and laboratory studies of ectopic humoral syndromes. Rec. Progr. Horm. Res. *25*, 283–314 (1969)
7. Mains, R. E., Eipper, B. A.: Coordinate synthesis of corticotropins and endorphins by mouse pituitary tumor cells. J. Biol. Chem. *253*, 651–655 (1978)

8. Meador, C. K., Liddle, G. W., Island, D. P., Nicholson, W. E., Lucas, C. P., Nuckton, J. G., Luetscher, J. A.: Cause of Cushing's syndrome in patients with tumors arising from "non endocrine" tissue. J. Clin. Endocrinol. Metab. *22,* 693–703 (1962)
9. Orth, D. N.: Adrenocorticotropic hormone (ACTH). In: Methods of Hormone Radioimmunoassay. Jaffe, B. M., Behrman, H. R. (eds.). New York: Academic Press 1978 (in press)
10. Orth, D. N., Guillemin, R., Ling, N., Nicholson, W. E.: Immunoreactive Endorphins, lipotropins and corticotropins in a human nonpituitary tumor: evidence for a common precursor. J. Clin. Endocrinol. Metab. *46,* 849–852 (1978)
11. Orth, D. N., Nicholson, W. E.: High molecular weight forms of human ACTH are glycoproteins. J. Clin. Endocrinol. Metab. *44,* 214–217 (1977)
12. Orth, D. N., Nicholson, W. E.: Different molecular forms of ACTH. Ann. N. Y. Acad. Sci. *297,* 27–48 (1977)
13. Orth, D. N., Nicholson, W. E., Mitchell, W. M., Island, D. P., Liddle, G. W.: Biologic and immunologic characterization and physical separation of ACTH and ACTH fragments in the ectopic ACTH syndrome. J. Clin. Invest. *52,* 1756–1769 (1973)
14. Orth, D. N., Tanaka, K., Nicholson, W. E.: Melanocyte stimulating hormones (MSH's) and lipotropic hormones (LPH's). In: Methods of Hormone Radioimmunoassay. Jaffe, B. M., Behrman, H. R. (eds.). New York: Academic Press 1978 (in press)
15. Ratcliffe, J. G., Scott, A. P., Bennett, H. P. J., Lowry, P. J., McMartin, C., Strong, J. A., Walbaum, P. R.: Production of a corticotrophin-like intermediate lobe peptide and of corticotrophin by a bronchial carcinoid tumour. Clin. Endocrinol. *2,* 51–55 (1973)
16. Rees, H. J., Ratcliffe, J. G.: Ectopic hormone production by non-endocrine tumours. Clin. Endocrinol. *3,* 263–299 (1974)
17. Roberts, J. L., Herbert, E.: Characterization of a common precursor to corticotropin and β-lipotropin: Identification of β-lipotropin peptides and their arrangement relative to corticotropin in the precursor synthesized in a cellfree system. Proc. Natl. Acad. Sci. USA. *74,* 5300–5304 (1977)
18. Rosen, S. W., Weintraub, B. D., Vaitukaitis, J. V., Sussman, H. H., Hershman, J. M., Muggia, F. M.: Placental proteins and their subunits as tumor markers. Ann. Intern. Med. *82,* 71–83 (1975)
19. Tanaka, K., Nicholson, W. E., Orth, D. N.: The nature of immunoreactive LPHs in human plasma and tissue extracts. J. Clin. Invest. (1978) (in press)
20. Yalow, R. S., Berson, S. A.: Size heterogeneity of immunoreactive human ACTH in plasma and in extracts of pituitary glands and ACTH-producing thymoma. Biochem. Biophys. Res. Commun. *44,* 439–445 (1971)

Prognostic Value of Postoperative Blood Levels of Carcinoembryonic Antigen (CEA) in Breast Cancer

R. E. Myers, D. J. A. Sutherland, J. W. Meakin, D. G. Malkin, J. A. Kellen, and A. Malkin

Introduction

Carcinoembryonic antigen (CEA) was originally described by GOLD in 1965. Initial studies suggested that this assay might provide a method for identifying patients with colon cancer. However, the early promise of specificity for colon cancer has not been confirmed by the antigen and antibody preparations currently available and, in fact, abnormally elevated levels of CEA have been found in a wide variety of tumours, other non-malignant diseases, and after blood transfusion. More refined antigen and antibody preparations hold promise of greater specificity [3].

With the relatively recent discovery that adjuvant chemotherapy and hormone therapy can reduce recurrence rates in premenopausal breast cancer patients, it becomes important to have means of selecting patients at high risk of recurrence. Traditionally, histological nodal status has served this function. Other tests of prognosis are required when the axillary nodes are negative. Furthermore, in patients with metastatic disease in particular, when one is comparing different treatment regimens, it is important to have means of assuring that different groups of patients are comparable.

At the Ontario Cancer Institute we have been measuring CEA levels in all new postoperative breast cancer patients referred to our hospital with the following aims:

1. To assess the percentage of patients with positive CEAs within different stages of breast cancer to see if it correlates with tumour burden;
2. To assess the value of a single postoperative CEA determination in predicting development of subsequent recurrent disease;
3. To assess the value of CEA as a prognostic factor in patients with metastatic disease.

This represents an interim report of our data.

Methods

In order to qualify for the study, patients were divided into primary cases and metastatic cases. In primary cases the CEA must have been performed less than or equal to 3 months after surgery. The patients must have had no evidence of residual or metastatic disease as determined by standard blood tests, scans and X-rays, and the CEA had to have been performed in a period between April 1975 and June 1976. All patients were staged according to UICC clinical staging criteria on the basis of the referring surgeon's description of the patient's tumour. Axillary node information was obtained from the pathologist's description of the tissue removed by the surgeon. The metastatic cases included any new patients who had metastatic disease at the time of registration at our hospital in whom a CEA was performed, plus a further group of patients with metastatic disease who had a CEA performed at a random time during their disease.

We have followed up both groups of patients until February 1978. The treatment of all these patients was decided on the basis of the clinical impression of the attending physician and not on the basis of the CEA value that was, in most cases, not available at the time the treatment decision was made.

The CEA levels were determined at Sunnybrook Hospital Medical Centre under the direction of one of us (A.M.) using the HANSEN assay [2] in which the 95th percentile for a normal female population was found to be 4.0 ng/ml. We have chosen a CEA of $\geq$ 4 ng/ml as representing an abnormal or elevated value. All graphs are actuarial. Statistical significance between graphs has been calculated using the Wilcoxan test [1]; otherwise, the chi-square and Fisher *t*-tests have been employed.

Results

CEA and Clinical Stage

Figure 1 presents the general distribution of all patients in this study as well as the numbers of patients in whom the CEA level was found to be elevated. It is seen that the percentage of elevated CEAs in postoperative breast cancer patients increased with stage: 15% in stage I, 23% in stage II, 20% in stage X (not stageable), and up to 40% in stage III patients. In the stage IV (patients with metastatic disease) 190/260 patients (73.1%) had elevated CEAs. These patients with metastatic disease will subsequently be analyzed separately from the primary cases.

Of the *total primary cases* in the second line of Fig. 1, 21.8% of the patients had elevated CEAs. When this group was further subdivided into *pathological nodal status,* as shown in the bottom line of Fig. 1, one finds that in the node-positive patients, 25.3% of patients had

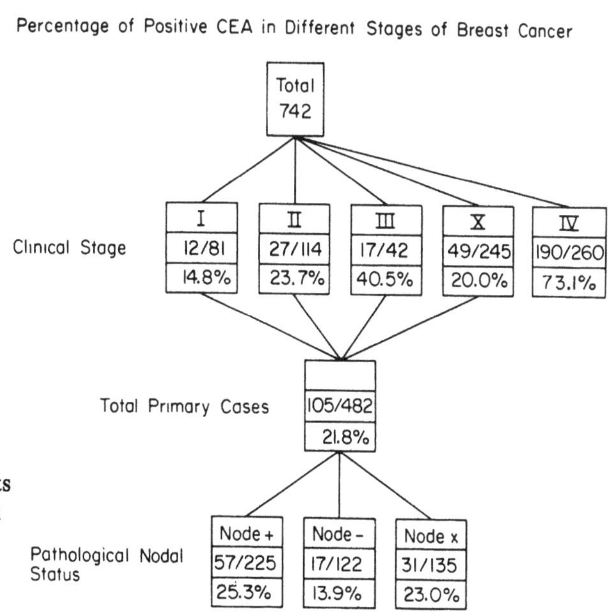

Fig. 1. The total number of patients and the percentage of patients with elevated CEAs are shown for each UICC stage and histological nodal category

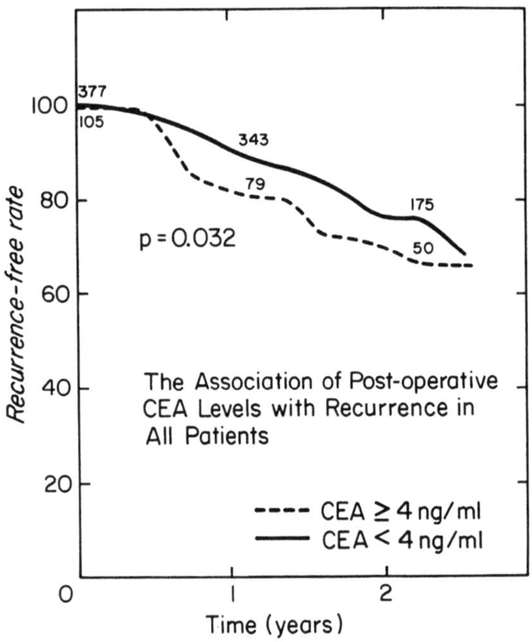

Fig. 2. Recurrence-free rate as a function of time from diagnosis for primary operable patients by level of postoperative plasma CEA levels. The numbers on top of the curves represent actual numbers followed to different time intervals

elevated CEAs compared to only 13.9% of the node-negative patients. In the node X (where nodal status was not known), CEAs were found to be elevated in 23% of cases.

We have now followed the primary cases for a mean period of 705 days from diagnosis. The association of postoperative CEA levels with recurrence for all operable patients is shown in Fig. 2. The numbers at the top of the curves represent the actual numbers of patients followed to a given time. From these graphs one can seen that the patients whose CEA is elevated tend to recur more quickly than their CEA-negative counterparts ($P = 0.03$), and indeed, at a year only 80% of the CEA-positive patients remained free of disease compared to almost 90% of the group who were CEA negative. However, with the passage of time, these differences become less marked and at 2½ years the curves appear to be coming together, which may be due to the small number of patients. The mean time to recurrence in the CEA-positive group was 362 days compared to 461 days in the CEA-negative group, a difference of almost 100 days ($P < 0.05$). This earlier recurrence in patients with elevated postoperative plasma CEA levels has been reflected in impaired survival, which is of borderline significance ($P = 0.07$).

Figure 3 shows the expected association of clinical stage with recurrence. Stage I, II and X patients (who demonstrated almost identical recurrence rates) have been combined and compared with stage III patients.

We attempted to analyze the importance of postoperative CEA levels within clinical stages and have found that, in patients with stages I, II and X disease, CEA values did not seem to play an important, predictive role in recurrence.

However, Fig. 4 shows the association of postoperative CEA levels with recurrence in stage III patients and here it is shown that, in patients who are CEA positive, at 2½ years only 20% remained disease free compared to almost 60% of patients who were CEA negative ($P = 0.05$).

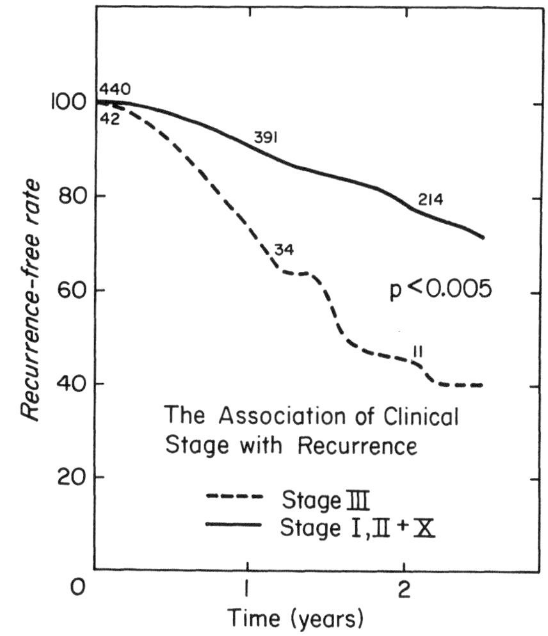

Fig. 3. Recurrence-free rate as a function of time from diagnosis by UICC stage. Date for stages I, II and X were so similar they were combined into one graph

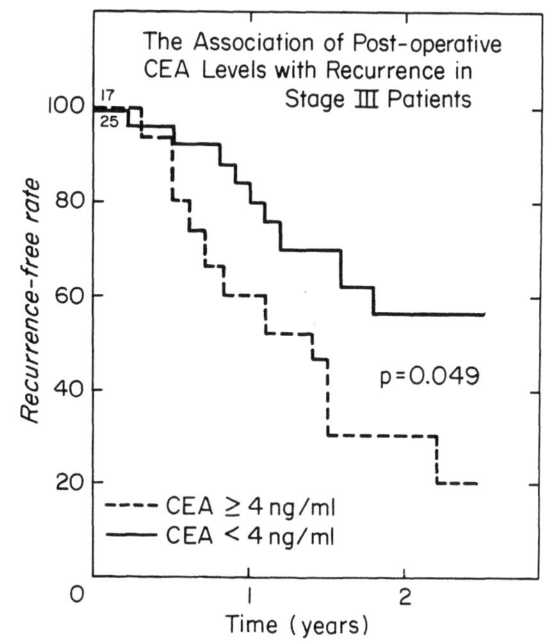

Fig. 4. Recurrence-free rate (Kaplan-Maier plot) as a function of time from diagnosis in stage III (UICC) patients by level of postoperative plasma CEA levels

CEA and Axillary Nodal Status

The well-known association of nodal status with recurrence after surgery is again demonstrated in Fig. 5. At 2½ years in the node-negative group, 80% remained disease free compared to only 65% in the node-positive group. We have attempted to analyze the

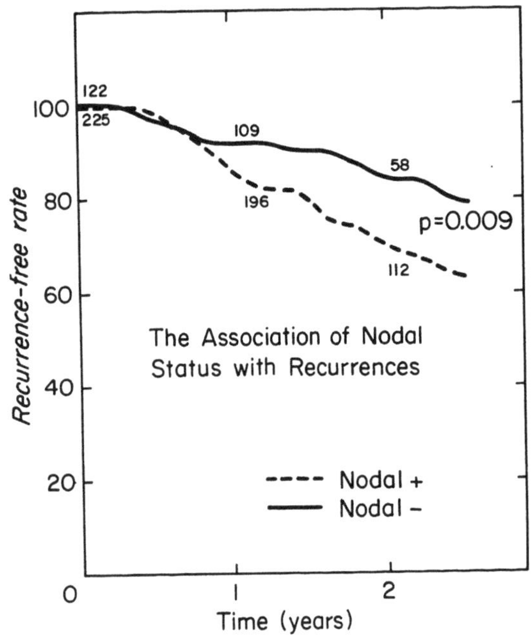

Fig. 5. Recurrence-free rate as a function of time from diagnosis in operable patients by axillary node histology

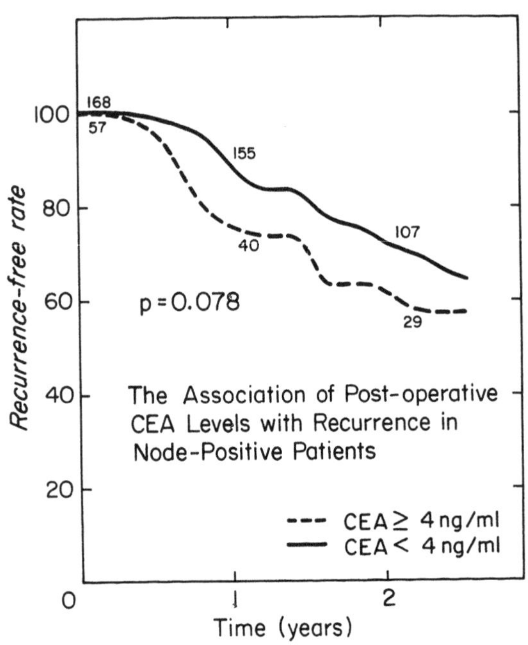

Fig. 6. Recurrence-free rate as a function of time from diagnosis in operable node-positive patients by postoperative plasma CEA levels

importance of postoperative CEA levels within nodal categories and have found that there appears, at this time, to be no prognostic importance of CEA levels in node-negative patients, which may be due to the small number (17, see Fig. 1) of node-negative patients that are CEA positive. However, the association of postoperative CEA levels with recurrence in node-positive patients is shown in Fig. 6. In the patients who are CEA positive, less than 60% are

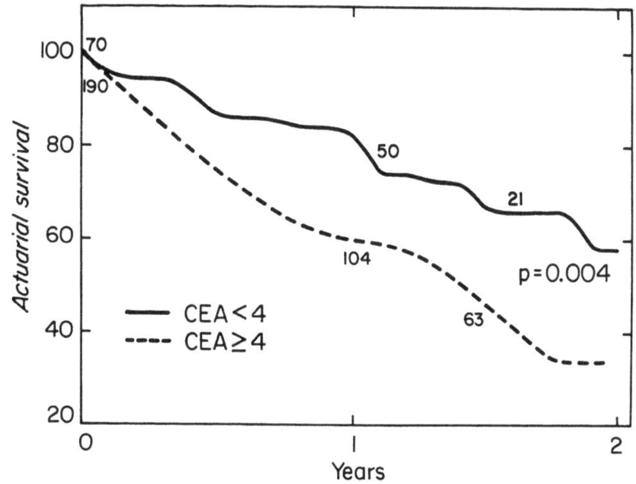

Fig. 7. Survival of patients with metastatic disease as a function of time from obtaining blood sample by plasma CEA level

disease free at 2½ years, compared to almost 70% of CEA-negative patients, but the difference is of borderline significance ($P = 0.08$).

CEA and Metastatic Disease

The prognostic significance of CEA values in 260 patients with metastatic disease is shown in Fig. 7. Survival has been measured from the date of CEA estimation. The patients have been followed a mean period of 256 days. There is a highly significant difference in survival. The patients whose CEAs are elevated have a median survival of 1.4 years, but the patients whose CEA is normal have not yet reached their median survival, which probably will be greater than 2 years. We have analyzed the two groups, CEA positive and negative, for extent and sites of disease and found no difference in tumour burden. However, bone metastases occurred in 52% of patients with elevated CEAs compared to 33% of patients with normal CEA values ($P = 0.01$). Visceral metastases occurred in 19% of CEA-positive patients compared to 38% of CEA-negative patients ($P = 0.008$).

Conclusions

The percentage of postoperative breast cancer patients having elevated plasma CEA values increases with UICC clinical stage. The presence of an elevated CEA in postoperative breast cancer patients is associated with a higher incidence of early recurrence than in patients where the CEA is normal, which is in agreement with previously published data [4, 5]; this effect may be independent of nodal status or clinical stage. The mean time to recurrence in CEA-positive patients was 100 days shorter than in those with normal values. Patients with metastatic disease in whom the CEA is found to be elevated have a distinctly inferior prognosis compared to those with normal values, which is not explainable on the basis of sites of metastases or tumour burden as measured by conventional means.

Acknowledgement

This study has been supported in part by the Ontario Cancer Treatment and Research Foundation.

References

1. Gehan, E. A.: A generalized Wilcoxon test for comparing arbitrarily singly-sensored samples. Biometrika *52,* 203–223 (1965)
2. Hansen, H. J., Snyder, J. J., Miller, E., Vandevoorde, J. P., Miller, O. N., Hines, L. R., Burns, J. J.: Carcinoembryonic antigen (CEA) assay. A laboratory adjunct in the diagnosis and management of cancer. Hum. Pathol. *5,* 139–147 (1974)
3. Maugh II, T. H.: CEA: Puzzling new information about a useful marker. Science *197,* 544 (1977)
4. Myers, R. E., Sutherland, D. J. A., Kellen, J. A., Malkin, D. G., Malkin, A.: CEA in breast cancer. Cancer (in press) (1978)
5. Wang, D. Y., Bulbrook, R. D., Hayward, J. L., Hendrick, J. C., Franchimont, P.: Relationship between plasma carcinoembryonic antigen and prognosis in women with breast cancer. Eur. J. Cancer *11,* 615–618 (1975)

α-Fetoprotein (αFP) as a Marker for Hepatoma and Yolk Sac Tumors

D. Buffe and C. Rimbaut

The α-1-fetoprotein is the first globulin to appear in mammalian serum during development, in very early embryonic and fetal life [2, 4, 6]. In serum, it reaches maximal concentration, about 4 mg/ml in the 12th–14the week of fetal age. After birth, its level falls rapidly, within a few weeks, to the adult level of 10–15 ng/ml.
In certain pathologic status, abnormal values have been observed. In 1963 Abelev noted the occurrence of the embryonic αFP in the serum of hepatoma-bearing mice [1]. One year later, Tatarinov reported one case of primary liver carcinoma with a abnormal level of αFP [11]. Since this period, many publications throughout the world have pointed out the diagnostic value of αFP for two types of tumors: primary liver carcinoma and teratocarcinoma with vitelline components [3, 7, 8, 9, 10].
The use of the very sensitive technique of radioimmunoassay has increased the prognostic value of the serum αFP detection, which has become a helpful tool in following the clinical course and in the detection of residual disease in patients with germ cell tumors and hepatoma. To confirm the clinical significance of αFP in residual tumors or recurrences, we now report some pathologic cases in which determination of the serum αFP level was able to indicate incomplete surgery or a recurrence, sometimes very early.

Case 1. A 4-year-old girl had a sacrococcygeal teratoma. The serum αFP level was very high (20 μg/ml). After surgery, this level decreased, but not sufficiently; 3 months later it was still above 1 μg/ml. This was an indication of incomplete excision (Fig. 1). It is well-known that the half-life of αFP is about 7–9 days: even if an abnormal blood αFP level is still observed for several days or weeks after surgery (depending on the initial presurgery level), it should fall to the normal level in less than 1 month to give a sure indication of complete surgical excision or cure. In this child a recurrence was quickly observed with a rising αFP level.

Case 2. An 18-month-old boy was found to have an enlargement of the right testis discovered after mumps. An exploratory orchidectomy was performed in August 1975. Histologic examination showed an embryonic tumor with vitelline components. The αFP level before operation is not known, but 1 month later it was 60 ng/ml (Fig. 2). A three-drug chemotherapy was given. The child was clinically well but there was no check on αFP for 9 months. At this time, the level of αFP was found to be 200 ng/ml. The raised αFP level was confirmed in another blood sample 3 weeks later. Radiography and lymphography seemed normal. Nevertheless, due to the αFP increase, an exploratory laparatomy was carried out, which showed metastatic lymph nodes. During this period, αFP was increasing and in spite of radio- and chemotherapy, the child died with lung and liver metastasis.

Case 3. A hepatoma was detected in a young man of 26 [5]. This man was admitted to hospital because of illhealth and digestive troubles. Painful hepatomegaly was observed. The αFP concentration was highly abnormal: 1250 μg/ml. The right lobe of the liver was resected and a large tumor (weight 2500 g) removed. The αFP was regularly monitored after surgery (Fig. 3) by means of a technique that detects only concentrations above 1 μg/ml. One year later

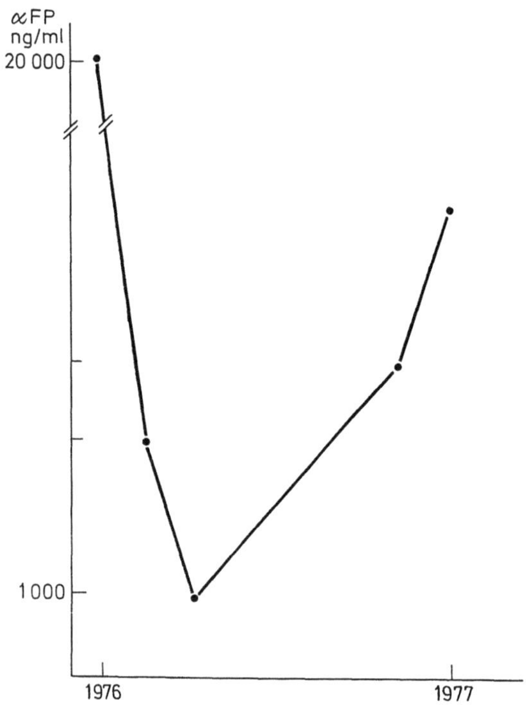

Fig. 1. Sacrococcygeal teratoma (case 1)

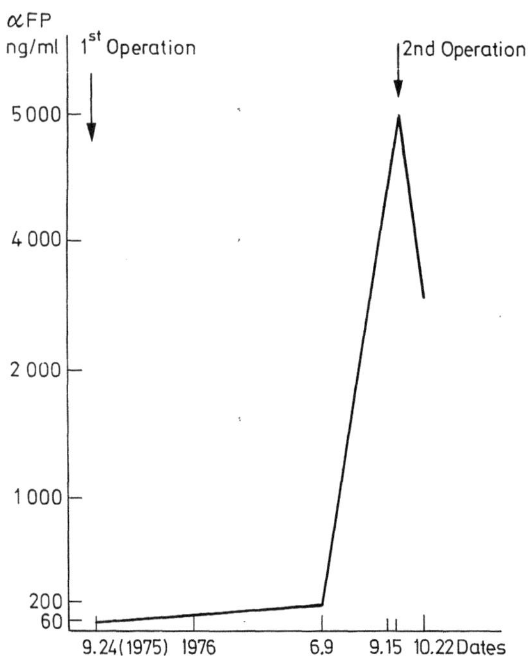

Fig. 2. Testis tumor (case 2)

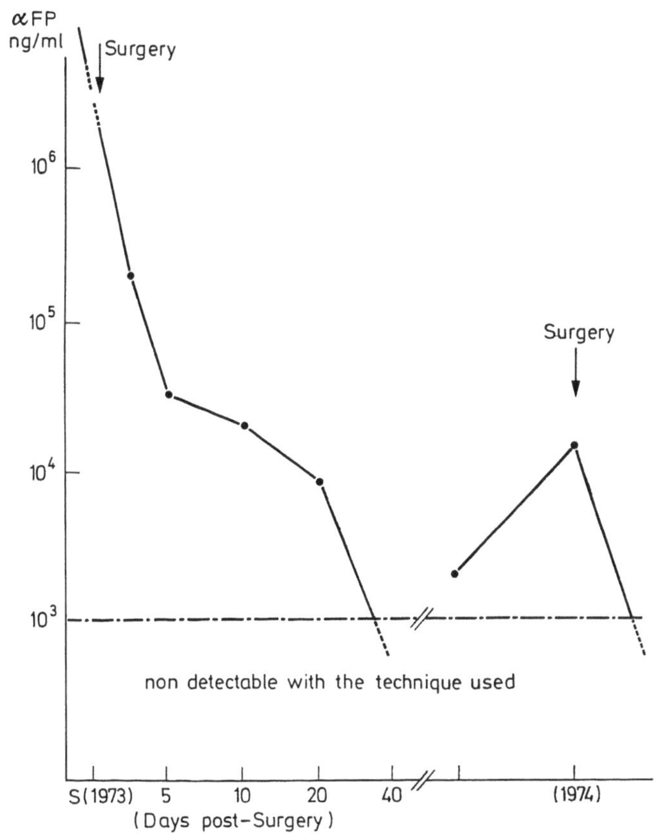

Fig. 3. Hepatoma (case 3)

(1973), the clinical state was good but blood examination revealed αFP levels of 2.5 μg/ml and 11 μg/ml 12 days later. Hepatic arteriography and scintigraphy were normal. A further surgical exploration was carried out because of the increased αFP level. The surgeon, after a careful examination, detected two small tumors, 3 mm and 10 mm, on the inferior part of the left lobe. After surgery, αFP decreased but it never reached the normal level. It was always above 70–80 ng/ml when assayed by radioimmunoassay (normal level is less than 10 ng/ml). Many blood samples were not tested with a sufficiently sensitive method until April 1977. At this time an αFP level of 1000 ng/ml was found. In spite of a normal scintigraphy, a third operation was performed and three small recurrences were discovered. After excision αFP decreased; the level became normal 1 month later and has remained normal up to now (June, 1978) (Fig. 4).

Case 4. An 18-month-old boy was found to have a testis yolk sac tumor. A test for αFP was positive but we do not known the exact level. Ten and 20 days after surgery, the αFP concentration had decreased to 120 and 65 ng/ml, respectively; but by day 40 the αFP level had increased to 75 ng/ml. This rise signified a recurrence (Fig. 5), which was rapidly confirmed. The boy underwent further surgery and curettage of a lymph gland was performed, after which the αFP level became normal.

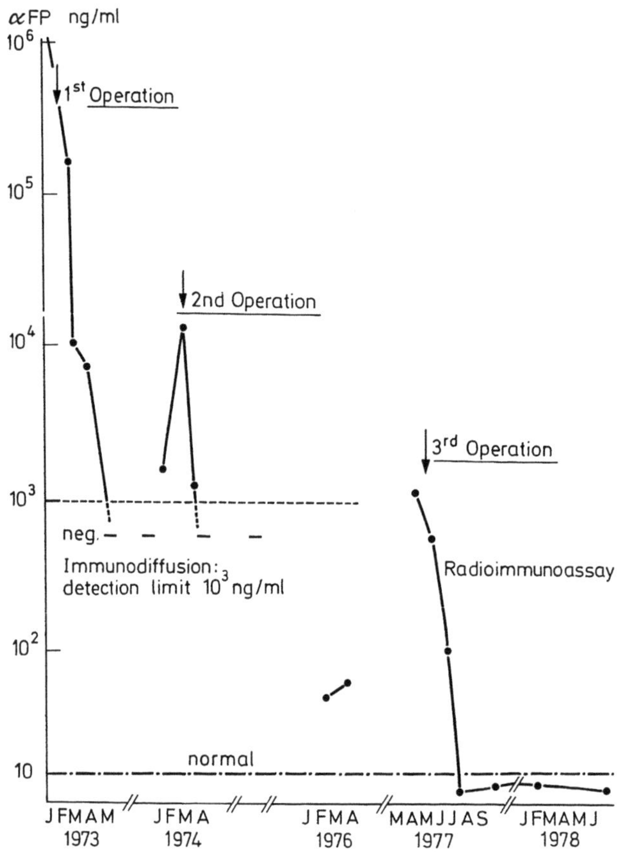

Fig. 4. Case 3 after excision

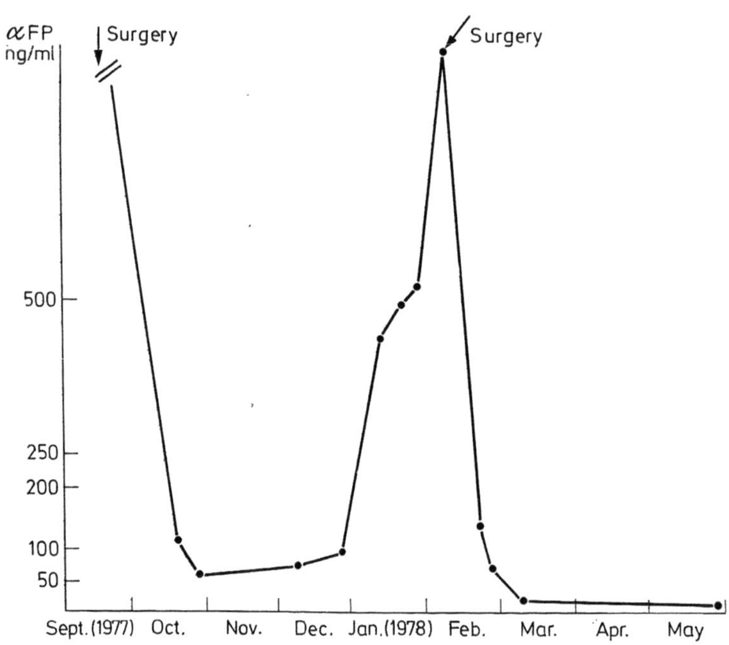

Fig. 5. Testis yolk sac tumor (case 4)

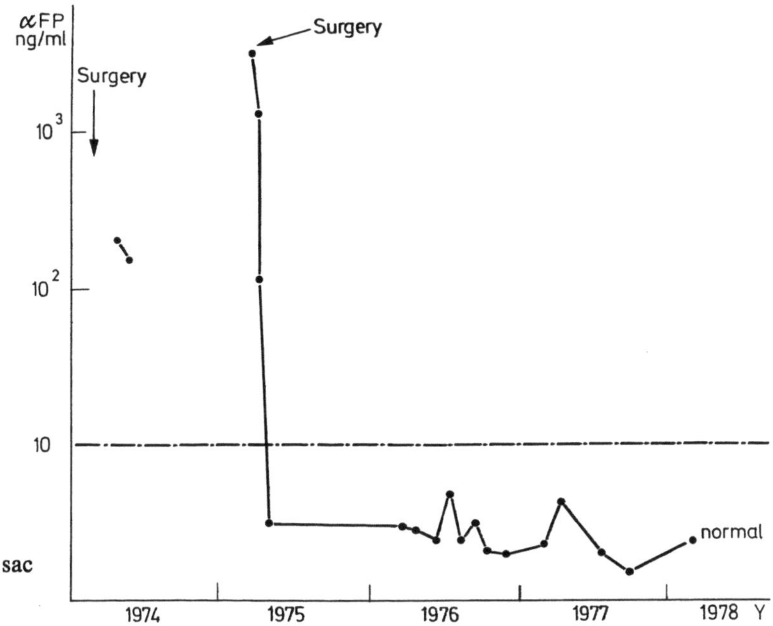

Fig. 6. Testis yolk sac tumor (case 5)

Case 5. A yolk sac tumor of the testis was detected in a 13 month old boy. At 6 months of age, a left testis enlargement was observed and a hydrocele testis was diagnosed. In 1974 an operation was performed and a tumor was discovered. The αFP, tested the day after surgery, was abnormal. It was still abnormal 3 weeks later, being over 200 ng/ml. Four courses of triple chemotherapy were given as an adjuvant, but the αFP was not monitored with any sensitive technique. A pulmonary metastasis was found 1 year later and the αFP rose to above 6 μg/ml. A thoracotomy was performed at which a tumor in the middle lobe and two diaphramatic metastases were removed. Hepatic scintigraphy was normal. The surgery was followed up with radio- and chemotherapy. The αFP level decreased quickly. It was inferior to 100 ng/ml in less than 1 month and inferior to 10 ng/ml in 2 months. All tests have since been normal (Fig. 6).

Conclusion

As demonstrated by these clinical studies, αFP is not only a valuable marker in the diagnosis of hepatocellular carcinoma and germ cell tumors containing vitelline components but also a useful tool for clinical follow-up of patients with these tumors and for very early detection of residual disease.

A persistently elevated αFP level in the serum after surgery indicates the presence of residual tumor or metastasis. Selective blood screening should be carried out in all patients with these types of tumors, according to the following schema, which has been derived from many observations:

1. One blood sample just before operations, to give a reference level;
2. one sample every 5–7 days in the post-surgery month;

3. one sample monthly during the 1st year;
4. one sample every 3 months during the 2nd year;
5. one sample every 6 months for the next 4 years.

Every sample should be tested with the same radioimmunoassay along with the original frozen and retained sample. An increase in the αFP level, even small, could be important. It should be quickly verified and clinical and surgical examinations must be performed to find its cause.

Acknowledgement

The clinical observation of case 3 is extracted from Dr. Didier Jacqumin's thesis.

References

1. Abelev, G. I., Perova, S. D., Khramkova, N. I., Postnikova, Z. A., Irlin, I. S.: Production of embryonal α globulin by transplantable mouse hepatomas. Transplantation *1*, 174–176 (1963)
2. Bergstrand, G. G., Czar, B.: Demonstration of new protein fraction in serum from human fetus. Scand. J. Clin. Lab. Invest. *8*, 174–177 (1956)
3. Buffe, D.: Les antigènes de tumeurs et leur détection dans le sérum: interet des méthodes radioimmunologiques. In: Radioimmunoassay and related procedures in medicine. International Atomic Energy Agency 1974 (ed.), Vol. II, pp. 253–265
4. De Muralt, G., Roulet, D. L. A.: Etude immunologique des proteines sériques foetales humaines. Helv. Peadiatr. Acta. *16*, 517–520 (1961)
5. Gallot, D., Hirsch Marie, H., Huguet, C., Caroli, J.: L'alpha foeto proteine (AFP) sérique après résection des cancers primitifs du foie chez l'adulte. Nouv. Presse Méd. *3*, 2305–2308 (1974)
6. Gitlin, D., Boesman, M.: Fetus specific serum proteins in several mammals and their relation to human α-1-Feto protein. Comp. Biochem. Physiol. *21*, 327–338 (1967)
7. Masseyeff, R. F.: Factors influencing α-1-Foeto protein biosynthesis in patients with primary liver cancer and other diseases. Gann (Monogr. Cancer Res.) *14*, 3–18 (1973)
8. O'Connor, G. T., Tatarinov, Y. S., Abelev, G. I., Uriel, J.: A collaborative study for the evaluation of a serologic test for primary liver cancer. Cancer *25*, 1091–1095 (1970)
9. Rimbaut, C., Caillaud, J. P., Caillou, B., Carlu, C., Rudant, C., Buffe, D.: Alpha-1-fetoprotein (AFP) and Germ Cell Tumors: Biological and Histological Correlation. 5th IRGCP Meeting of Int. Research Group for carcinoembryonic proteins "recent progress". Copenhagen, August (1977) (in press Scand. J. Immunol. *7*, Suppl. 8 (1978))
10. Smith, T. B.: Alpha fetoprotein: occurence in certain malignant diseases and review of clinical applications. Med. Clin. North Am. *54*, 797–802 (1970)
11. Tatarinov, Y. S.: Presence of embryo specific α globulin in the serum of patients with primary hepatocellular carcinoma. Vol. Med. Khim. *10*, 90–95 (1964)

Casein and Breast Cancer[1]

J. C. Hendrick, P. F. Zangerle, and P. Franchimont

The proteins of skim milk may be divided into two categories:
1. The milk-specific proteins, which predominate;
2. The proteins of plasma origin.

Caseins are the main components in the protein group of plasma origin. This group of phosphoproteins has an average concentration of 0.4 g per 100 ml of mature milk. Caseins appear as aggregates of calcium caseinate, and the turbidity of skim milk is due to this micellar dispersion. One can precipitate the caseins by acidification at pH 4.6 or by cold ultracentrifugation. Originally the different casein fractions were defined on the basis of their electrophoretic mobilities at alkaline pH. α-, β-, and γ-caseins were described, but chemical electrophoretic and chromatographic improvements indicated the existence of many other subfractions. It is now probable that caseins are the molecular variant of a single type of protein molecules phosphorylated at different levels.

In the method of Groves and Gordon [1], caseins are precipitated from skim milk at pH 4.6 and submitted to chromatography on DEAE cellulose. All the different protein peaks are obtained by stepwise elution as shown in Fig. 1. The hormonal dependance of some breast cancers and the intracellular secretary products suggest the synthesis of milk-like substances. It was then proposed that some mammary carcinomas could produce milk antigens. We have tried to clarify the problem of caseins in human breast cancer. With this objective we initiated radioimmunoassays of caseins in 1973 [2].

Our first results were obtained with a system using whole casein as tracer and standard. Antiserum was raised against whole casein. The sensitivity was poor: 100 ng/ml. Figure 2 shows the results in noncancerous patients. Some normal subjects showed abnormally elevated values up to 500 ng/ml and lactating women showed very elevated values up to 3000 ng/ml. In Fig. 3, results obtained for patients with carcinoma are shown. Positive results were obtained in many cases, even in lung and digestive cancers.

As this system was inadequate because of the presence of false positive values (up to 500 ng/ml) and because the tracers lacked stability, we decided to use purified subfractions of casein. K-Casein was then used as tracer and standard because of its better stability, but we continued to use the same antiserum as before. The sensitivity was then in the range of 10 ng/ml, and it was possible to test the cross reactivity of the different fractions of casein as shown in Fig. 4. Cross reactivity was complete between κ-caseins I and II but incomplete with caseins III and IV.

κ-casein levels were studied in the serum of benign and malignant mastopathy as shown in Fig. 5. The incidence of positivity (values higher then 25 ng/ml) was lower than previously described: 15% at the onset of clinical symptoms, 44% in the case of metastases [3], and 11% after surgical removal of the tumor. In all cases, the major immunoreactive peak was

1 Supported by grant 20305 of "Fonds de la Recherche Scientifique médicale (FRSM)" and by the "Fonds Cancérologique de la Caisse Générale d'Epargne et de Retraite," Belgium.

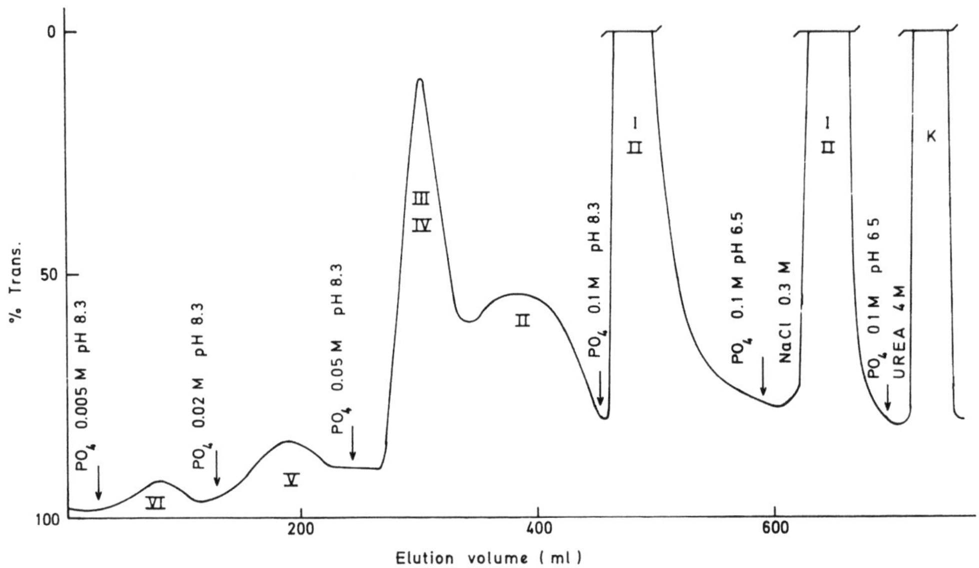

Fig. 1. Chromatography of caseins on DEAE cellulose

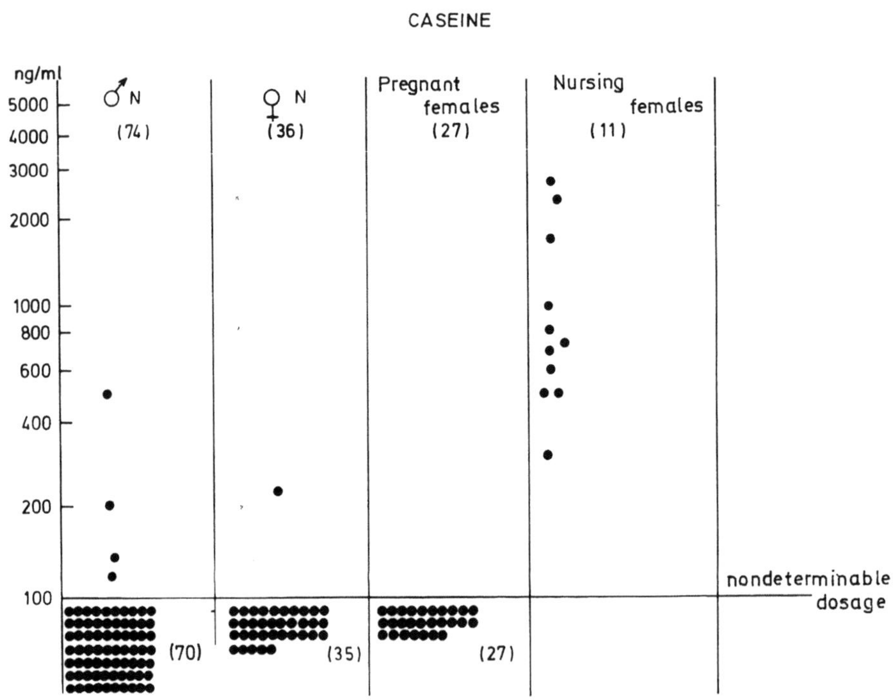

Fig. 2. Casein levels in noncancerous patients

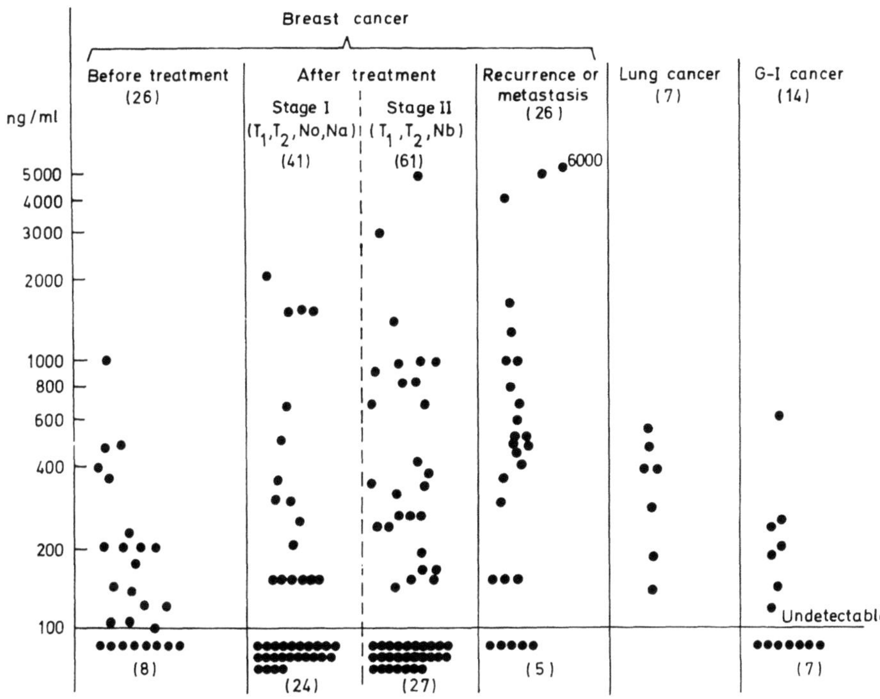

Fig. 3. Casein levels in patients with various malignancies

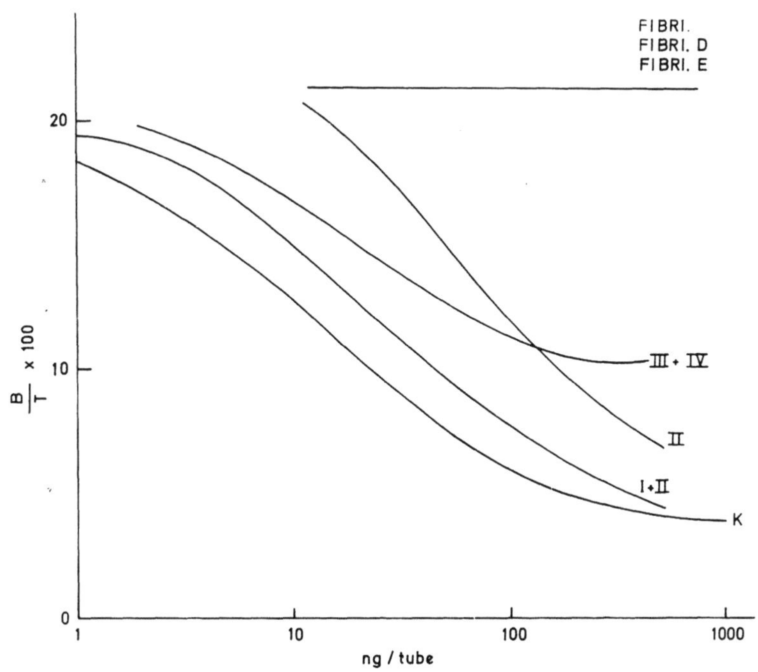

Fig. 4. Displacement curves using κ-casein (I + II, II, III + IV), intact fibrinogen, and fragments D and E of fibrinogen

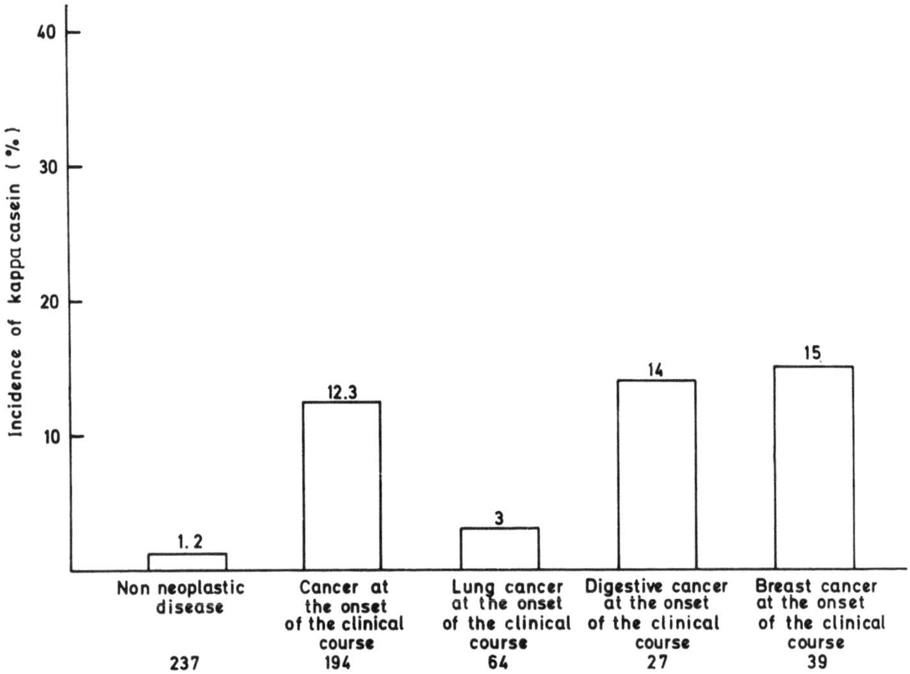

Fig. 5. κ-casein levels in the serum of benign and malignant mastopathy

displaced toward the lower molecular weight elution regions. Very often we found several peaks indicating a high degree of heterogeneity.

Additionally, we performed gel filtration of casein-rich sera on Sephadex G-200 column (2.5 × 30 cm) [exclusion volume was 54 ml, 2 ml of sample were applied, and optical density (280 nm) was measured for each fraction]. Casein content was estimated by radioimmunoassay [3]. Casein-like material present in the serum of cancerous patients showed a heterogenous elution pattern and in some cases a large spectrum of molecular weight (Fig. 6).

Attempts were made to obtain specific antisera directed against the different fractions of casein. It was possible to obtain a specific assay of κ-casein with no cross reaction with the other fractions. But in contrast, κ-casein was able to cross-react in a system using casein II as tracer and an antiserum directed against casein II. When these highly specific systems were used to detect casein in blood of noncancerous and cancerous patients, the incidence of positivity using only one system decreased, some sera being positive in one system and not in the others [5].

As we very often observed broad variations of normal and control values in the assay of casein, we wanted to known if the micellar nature of casein could explain this phenomenum. Blood samples were again chromatographed on Sephadex G-200: a first group in phosphate buffer, a second group in phosphate buffer plus 6 *M* urea (after pretreatment with 6 *M* urea), and a third group in buffer plus 6 *M* urea and 1% mercaptoethanol. The elution tubes were pooled in three classes: macroglobulin zone, γ-g zone, and albumin zone. They were carefully

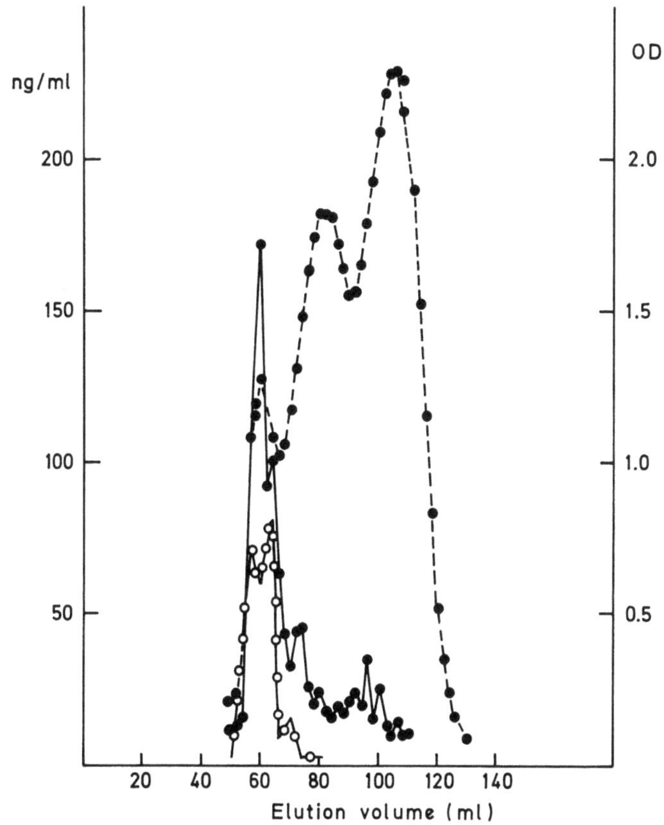

Fig. 6. Chromatography of serum from cancerous patients ○——○, ●——●, casein content; O.D

dialized against normal buffer. κ-Casein and casein II were tried (Fig. 7). It was obvious that the treatment with 6 *M* urea dismantled the micellar structure of casein and considerably increased the amount of immunologically active sites. The effect was more marked for casein II than for κ-casein. The use of 1% mercaptoethanol did not improve the phenomenum, certainly because this treatment was too drastic and destroyed the molecules.

This last experiment may indicate why the radioimmunoassay gives variable results. We believe that techniques of blood collection, the incubation mixture and temperature can all affect the micellar structure of caseins and perturbate the assay. Moreover, different antigenic sites are available on the different subunits. The circulating antigens show polymorphism: we never detected in the blood of lactating or cancerous women the monomeric form of the casein subfractions. It appears that a very high specificity of the assay is not useful for clinical application since the incidence of positivity is then decreased. It is dangerous to extrapolate the results obtained with one given subfraction and one particular antiserum to comment on the results obtained in other systems [4]. This complicated situation is interesting from the immunochemical point of view but makes the task very difficult for clinical purposes.

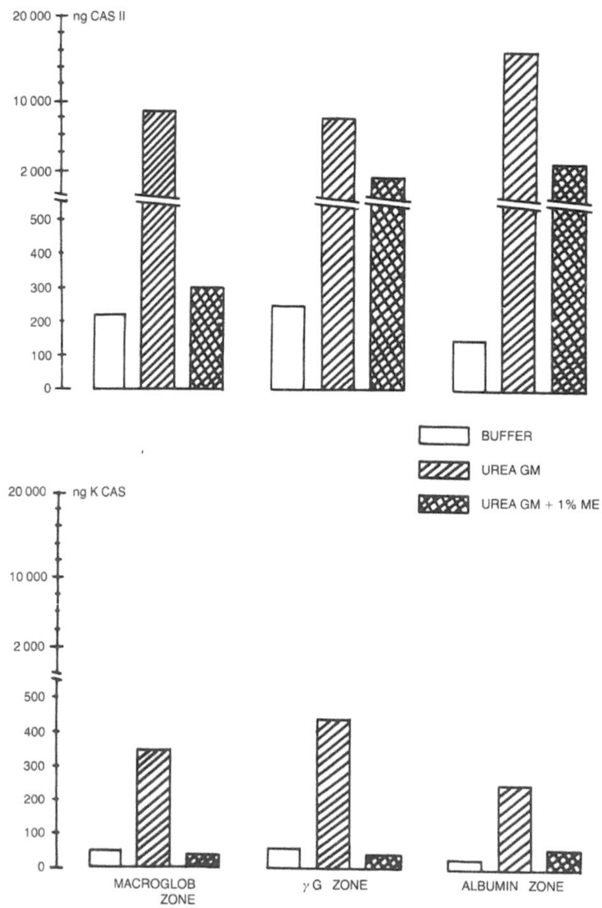

Fig. 7. κ-casein and casein II levels in eluted fractions from chromatographid serum under nondissociating and dissociating conditions

References

1. Groves, M. L., Gordon, W. G.: The major component of human casein. A protein phosphorylate at different levels. Arch. Biochem. *140,* 47 (1970)
2. Hendrick, J. C., Franchimont, P.: Radioimmunoassay of casein in the serum of normal subjects and of patients with various malignancies. Eur. J. Cancer *10,* 725 (1974)
3. Hendrick, J. C., Thirion, A., Franchimont, P.: Radioimmunoassay of casein. In: Cancer related antigens. Franchimont, P. (ed.), p. 51. Amsterdam: Elsevier North Holland 1976
4. Monaco, M. E., Bronzert, D. A., Tormey, D. C., Waalkes, P., Lippman, M. E.: Casein production by human breast cancer. Cancer Res. *37,* 749 (1977)
5. Zangerle, P. F., Hendrick, J. C., Thirion, A., Franchimont, P.: Casein radioimmunoassay as an index of mammary function and as a tumor marker. In: Cancer related antigens. Franchimont, P. (ed.), pp. 61. Amsterdam: Elsevier North Holland 1976

Prostatic Acid Phosphatase and Prostatic Cancer

A. G. Foti, J. F. Cooper, and H. Herschman

Prostatic acid phosphatase (PAP, EC 3.1.3.2) is a specific acid phosphatase derived from the prostate gland. In normal males a small but detectable level of this enzyme is present in serum. When PAP was found to be elevated in the serum of patients with prostatic cancer [2, 3, 14, 17], the measurement of this enzyme became an accepted clinical adjunct in the detection and diagnosis of prostatic malignancy.

PAP activity is found in several isoenzymes. The separation of isoenzymes was first accomplished on starch gel electrophoresis by Sur et al. [22]. The concentration of PAP in prostatic tumors is about 8%–12% of that found in normal prostatic tissue. Several investigators have separated two isoenzymes from benign hyperplastic prostatic tissue [12, 18, 25]. We have separated two major PAP isoenzymes from both normal and cancerous prostatic tissue on DEAE cellulose columns, by isoelectric focusing, and by electrophoresis on polyacrylamide gel. However, apart from the difference in their ratio, there is no evidence, to date, of the existence of any qualitative differences between the two PAP isoenzymes found in normal and cancerous prostatic tissue [12].

When a tumor is confined to the prostatic capsule (stages I and II), treatment results in a 60%–70% 5-year survival rate [15]. In the later stages of the disease (stages III and IV), the tumor extends beyond the prostatic capsule and spreads to the lymph nodes and bone. For this group, the 5-year survival rate is less than 25% [4]. Thus, early detection, of prostatic cancer, followed by aggressive therapy, should result in a significantly reduced mortality rate for this disease.

Measurement of the concentration of serum PAP by the current enzymatic assay procedure has not been very effective in the early recognition of prostatic cancer, i.e., at the point when the tumor is still confined to the prostatic capsule [8]. There are many possible reasons for the enzyme assay's insufficiency, such as the instability of PAPs enzymatic activity at higher temperatures and the enzyme's susceptibility to denaturation upon changes in pH [11, 26]. In addition, the substrates used to measure PAP react with other acid phosphatases of nonprostatic origin. The measurement of PAP by enzyme assay, therefore, requires the introduction of inhibitors to increase the test's specificity [1, 16]. The assay's reliance on this type of indirect measurement of PAP considerably decreases the test's quantitative accuracy.

We have begun to use immunologic procedures for the measurement of serum PAP to circumvent the problems encountered in the enzyme assay and, hopefully, to improve the detection of prostatic cancer in its early stages [5, 19]. The antigen was purified from prostatic fluid and antiserum was raised in rabbits. After precipitation of the nonspecific antibodies with normal female serum, our antiserum appeared to be monospecific for serum PAP [10]. Several immunologic methods were considered for the quantitation of the antigen-antibody complex, including double diffusion [21], immunoelectrophoresis [13], counterimmunoelectrophoresis [9], complement fixation [23], and radioimmunoassay [5]. However, only the radioimmunoassay was found to be sensitive enough to measure the concentration of serum PAP in normal males, thereby enabling the establishment of a normal range of values [9, 10].

We developed and currently use a solid-phase radioimmunoassay for the measurement of serum PAP [10]. A diluted antiserum solution (1 : 3000) is used to coat the walls of a polypropylene vial. After removal of the antiserum solution, bovine serum albumin is used to saturate the remaining protein binding sites on the plastic wall. The incubation mixture consists of buffer, serum sample or PAP standard, and ^{125}I-labeled PAP. After a 36-h incubation, the free ^{125}I antigen is removed by aspiration and washing, and the amount of radioactivity remaining bound to the vial is determined. In our laboratory, one technician can evaluate 150 patients, in duplicate, in about 8 h, excluding the incubation time.

The immunologic reactivity of PAP antibody with extracts from various normal tissues has been measured by this method and less than 1% cross reactivity was found [10]. A comparison of the heat stability of serum PAP using the enzymatic assay and the radioimmunoassay demonstrated that while the enzyme activity of serum PAP begins to decrease after 1 h at room temperature, the immunologic activity of serum PAP is stable for over 48 h, at the serum pH of 8.2 [11].

We performed a randomized study to compare the ability of the enzyme assay and the radioimmunoassay for serum PAP to detect prostatic cancer in patients with different stages of the disease. Sera from 50 normal males, 113 untreated prostatic cancer patients (24 stage I, 33 stage II, 31 stage III, 25 stage IV), 36 patients with benign prostatic hyperplasia, 28 patients with total prostatectomy, 83 patients with cancers at other primary sites, and 20 patients with various gastrointestinal diseases were utilized in this study. The serum samples were randomized and coded, and the serum PAP level of all samples was measured by both enzyme assay and radioimmunoassay. After all analyses were completed and samples were designated as "normal" or "elevated," the code was broken. In this study, 33%, 79%, 71%, and 92% of stage I, II, III, and IV prostatic cancer cases, respectively, were correctly classified by radioimmunoassay. The enzyme assay detected 12%, 15%, 29%, and 60% of the same patients. Thus, the radioimmunoassay was able to correctly classify considerably more cases of intracapsular prostatic cancer than the enzymatic assay for PAP [8].

In the past 3 years we have utilized the radioimmunoassay for serum PAP to evaluate over 8000 patients, including both normal males and females and those with a variety of diseases. Approximately 3%–5% of the assayed serum samples showed falsely elevated levels of serum PAP, a somewhat larger proportion than that found with the enzyme assay. The largest single group with falsely increased concentrations of serum PAP were patients with bronchogenic malignancies; 20%–30% of this group had abnormally high levels of serum PAP by radioimmunoassay, regardless of their sex. It should be noted that the majority of these patients also exhibited elevated concentrations of serum PAP by enzyme assay [8].

The measurement of PAP from bone marrow has been suggested as a potential aid to clinicians in staging prostatic cancer and thus as an aid in selecting the appropriate treatment. However, the reliability of the quantitation of bone marrow PAP by enzyme assay is a very controversial subject [7, 24]. Many investigators have shown that the interference of other acid phosphatases present in bone marrow results in a very high proportion of false positive results when the enzyme assay is used. In contrast, after evaluating over 200 patients with the radioimmunoassay for bone marrow PAP, we have found that the results of the radioimmunoassay correlate well with the findings of the patient's bone scans and bone marrow pathology, without an unacceptably high percentage of false positives [6].

In several of our clinical cases, a patient diagnosed as having stage I or stage II prostatic cancer, on the basis of negative bone scans and staging pelvic lympadenectomy, began receiving supervoltage radiotherapy. However, after 6–12 months of increasing bone pain, a repetition of the bone scan revealed bony metastasis. The micrometastases had not been detected by the original bone scans. Our introduction of the radioimmunoassay to the evaluation of bone marrow PAP has made possible the detection of many micrometastases before they were detectable by bone scan. This institution (Kaiser Foundation Hospital), therefore, routinely evaluates the concentration of bone marrow PAP in patients with presumptive stage II and stage III disease before they receive treatment.

Our preliminary data suggest that sequential monitoring of PAP levels by radioimmunoassay, during and after a specific course of treatment, can provide the clinician with useful information as to the therapeutic effect of the treatment. An increased level of serum PAP is usually an indication of the recurrence of disease. Drugs that are used for the treatment of cancer patients do not interfere with the accuracy of the radioimmunoassay. However, rectal examination, sigmoidoscopy, or any other manipulation of the prostate gland increases the concentration of serum PAP (Table 1). Therefore, we recommend that blood for the determination of PAP by radioimmunoassay not be drawn within 24 h after such procedures.

We are presently engaged in a study to evaluate the radioimmunoassay for PAP as a screening test for prostatic cancer (Table 2). In the last 5 months, 4351 males, over the age of 50, from our outpatient clinic were evaluated. Blood was drawn randomly and, if the

Table 1. The effect of transurethral resection of the prostate on the concentration of serum prostatic acid phosphatase

Patient No.	Diagnosis	Prostatic acid phosphatase (ng/0.1 ml serum)			
		Preoperative	Midoperative	Postoperative	48 h
2726	BPH	3.1	7.7	108.0	–
2993	CaP (stage III)	10.6	35.0	70.0	9.4
2248	CaP (stage IV) bone met.	13.3	16.8	17.5	14.8

Normal range: 1.5–6.5 ng/0.1 ml serum.

Table 2. Initial results of the prostatic screening project

Number of patients screened	4351
Number of elevated samples	247
Number of known cancers	23
Stage I	1
Stage II	7
Stage III	10
Stage IV	5
Number of patients seen by a urologist:	41
Confirmed cancer	5
Suspicious	15
BPH	18

radioimmunoassay showed abnormally high levels of serum PAP, the patient's chart was consulted in order to exclude those patients who had had a rectal examination within 24 h of the blood test. Out of 247 patients who demonstrated elevated levels of serum PAP, 23 were known prostatic cancer patients and had been treated with some type of therapy; one patient had stage I, seven patients had stage II, ten patients had stage III, and five patients had stage IV prostatic cancer. Forty-three patients out of the remaining 222 were examined by a urologist; 15 were found to be suspicious by rectal examination and were referred for further work-up, and 18 of the men seen by a urologist were diagnosed, after rectal examination, as having benign prostatic hyperplasia (BPH). It appears that patients with BPH over 100 g show elevated levels of serum PAP. Out of nine patients who had further examination and complete work-up, including biopsy, open surgery, bone scan, etc., two were found to have stage II, two stage III, and one stage IV prostatic carcinoma. For the remaining four patients, the work-up resulted in no positive identification of prostatic cancer.

The radioimmunoassay for serum PAP thus provides an improved method for detecting early prostatic carcinoma, and its extension to the measurement of bone marrow PAP enables considerably more accurate staging of prostatic cancer patients with metastatic bone lesions than was previously possible.

Acknowledgement

Supported in part by contract CA 23667-01 from the National Cancer Institute and by a contract (EY-76-C-03-0012) between the Department of Energy and the Regents of the University of California.

We express our sincere appreciation to Sarah Sapon for her assistance.

References

1. Abul-Fadl, M. A. M., King, E. J.: Properties of the acid phosphatases of erythrocytes and of the human prostate gland. Biochem. J. *45*, 51–60 (1949)
2. Bodansky, A.: Phosphatase studies. II. Determination of serum phosphatase. Factors influencing the accuracy of the determination. J. Biol. Chem. *101*, 93–104 (1933)
3. Bonner, C. D., Homburger, F., Smithy, G. B.: "Prostatic" serum acid phosphatase level in cancer of the prostate. J. Am. Med. Assoc. *164*, 1070–1076 (1957)
4. Catalona, W. J., Scott, W. W.: Carcinoma of the prostate: A review. J. Urol. *119*, 1–8 (1978)
5. Cooper, J. F., Foti, A. G.: A radioimmunoassay for prostatic acid phosphatase: 1. Methodology and range of normal male serum values. Invest. Urol. *12*, 98–102 (1974)
6. Cooper, J. F., Foti, A. G., Shank, P. W.: Radioimmunochemical measurement of bone marrow acid phosphatase. J. Urol. *119*, 392–395 (1978)
7. Dias, S. R., Barnett, R. N.: Elevated bone marrow acid phosphatase: The problem of false positives. J. Urol. *117*, 749–751 (1977)
8. Foti, A. G., Cooper, J. F., Herschman, H., Malvaez, R. R.: Detection of prostatic cancer by solid-phase radioimmunoassay of serum prostatic acid phosphatase. New Engl. J. Med. *297*, 1357–1361 (1977)
9. Foti, A. G., Cooper, J. F., Herschman, H.: Counterimmunoelectrophoresis in determination of prostatic acid phosphatase in human serum. Clin. Chem. *24*, 140–142 (1978)

10. Foti, A. G., Herschman, H., Cooper, J. F.: A solidphase radioimmunoassay for human prostatic acid phosphatase. Cancer Res. *35,* 2446–2452 (1975)
11. Foti, A. G., Herschman, H., Cooper, J. F.: Comparison of human prostatic acid phosphatase by measurement of enzymatic activity and by radioimmunoassay. Clin. Chem. *23,* 95–99 (1977)
12. Foti, A. G., Herschman, H., Cooper, J. F.: Isozymes of acid phosphatase in normal and cancerous human prostatic tissue. Cancer Res. *37,* 4120–4124 (1977)
13. Grabar, P., Williams, C. A.: Methode immuno-electrophoretique d'analyse de melanges de substances antigeniques. Biochim. Biophys. Acta *17,* 67–74 (1955)
14. Gutman, A. B., Gutman, E. B.: An "acid" phosphatase occurring in the serum of patients with metastasizing carcinoma of the prostate gland. J. Clin. Invest. *17,* 473–478 (1938)
15. Heise, H. W.: Cancers of the male genital organs. In: Cancer patient survival 5. Axtell, L. M. et al. (eds.), pp. 190–196. Bethesda (Maryland): U.S. Dept. of Health, Education, and Welfare, Public Health Service, National Institutes of Health, National Cancer Institute 1976
16. Jacobsson, K.: The determination of tartrate-inhibited phosphatase in serum. J. Clin. Lab. Invest. *12,* 367–380 (1960)
17. Kent, J. R., Hill, M., Bischoff, A.: Acid phosphatase content of prostatic exprimate from patients with advanced prostatic carcinoma: A potential prognostic and therapeutic index. Cancer *25,* 858–862 (1970)
18. Mattila, S.: Detection of two molecular forms of the human prostatic acid phosphatase. Invest. Urol. *6,* 337–344 (1969)
19. Moncure, C. W., Johnston, C. L., Jr., Koontz, W. W., Jr., Smith, M. J. V.: Investigation of specific antigens in prostatic cancer. Cancer Chemotherap. Rep. (Part I) *59,* 105–110 (1975)
20. Murphy, G. P., Reynoso, G., Kenny, G. M., Gaeta, J. F.: Comparison of total and prostatic fraction serum acid phosphatase levels in patients with differentiated and undifferentiated prostatic carcinoma. Cancer *23,* 1309–1314 (1969)
21. Ouchterlony, O.: Diffusion in gel methods for immunological analysis. Prog. Allergy *5,* 1–78 (1958)
22. Sur, B. K., Moss, D. W., King, E. J.: Starch-gel electrophoresis of prostatic acid phosphatase. Proc. Assoc. Clin. Biochem. *2,* 11–13 (1962)
23. Taranta, A., Franklin, E. C.: Complement fixation by antibody fragments. Science *134,* 1981–1982 (1961)
24. Veenema, R. J., Gursel, E. O., Romas, N., Wechsler, M., Latimer, J. K.: Bone marrow acid phosphatase: Prognostic value in patients undergoing radical prostatectomy. J. Urol. *117,* 81–82 (1977)
25. Vihko, P., Kontturi, M., Korhonen, L. K.: Purification of human prostatic acid phosphatase by affinity chromatography and isoelectric focusing. Part I. Clin. Chem. *24,* 466–470 (1978)
26. Woodard, H. Q.: A note on the inactivation by heat of acid glycerophosphatase in alkaline solution. J. Urol. *65,* 688–690 (1951)

Sialyl Transferase Activity: A Serum Enzyme Marker in the Follow-Up of Cancer Patients

U. Ganzinger and K. Moser

Introduction

Changed activities of glycosyl transferases are thought to correlate with malignant degeneration of cells. This was found by examination of serum samples of cancer patients [1, 9, 10]. Particular importance is attached to one specific glycosyl transferase, namely sialyl transferase. This enzyme incorporates "activated" sialic acid into appropriate acceptors. Sialic acid is frequently found in glycoproteins and glycolipids as a terminal sugar residue. It has been demonstrated by our group and others that sialyl transferase shows greater activity in the serum or plasma of cancer patients than in that of normal healthy subjects [2–5]. Preliminary results in the diagnosis of malignant disease by means of this enzyme determination so far allow the following conclusions to be drawn:

1. There is a strong correlation between tumor extent and enzyme activity. Patients with large tumor masses, whether large primary tumors or extensive metastases, have considerably higher enzyme values than patients with small tumors. This applies not only for breast and colon cancer, but also for Hodgkin's disease [6, 7];
2. Reduction or removal of tumor tissue, e.g., surgically, results in a significant decrease of enzyme activity. According to the clinical state of primary cancers, the enzyme activity before surgery is evidently increased over that of normal healthy subjects. After surgery

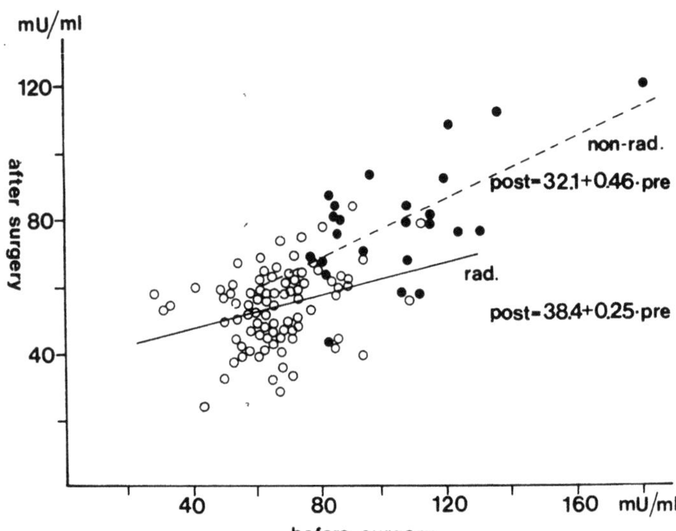

Fig. 1. Influence of surgical tumor removal on serum sialyl transferase activity. In both groups (radical and nonradical surgery) there is a significant ($P < 0.001$) decrease in enzyme activity after surgery. Radical: 68.1 ± 13.7 → 55.2 ± 11.5 mU/ml; Nonradical: 102.2 ± 17.7 → 80.9 ± 17.4 mU/ml

Table 1. Serum sialyl transferase activity in patients with or without relapses

	Breast cancer		Gastrointestinal cancer		Various cancers	
	meta.	no rel.	meta.	no rel.	meta.	no rel.
Over 74.8 mU/ml	71	21	21	8	42	5
Below 74.8 mU/ml	25	91	7	42	15	17
Over 74.8 mU/ml	$\chi^2 = 61.66$		$\chi^2 = 24.29$		$\chi^2 = 15.06$	
Below 74.8 mU/ml	$P < 0.001$		$P < 0.001$		$P < 0.001$	
$CC_{corr.}$	0.676		0.689		0.566	

Meta.: metastases, no rel.: no relapses. The number of patients examined is shown. Per patient only one value was taken, if there were several values the highest was used and correlated with clinical course of the appropriate day.

there is a significant decrease in the enzyme activity, in the radical-surgery group mostly back to normal range. After nonradical surgery the value is also significantly lowered but not to the normal range. One reason for this is residual tumor tissue (Fig. 1);

3. Enzyme activity increases in patients with tumor burden to the same extent as it is lowered in patients with undetectable tumor masses after a radical operation. A total of 74% of patients examined with proved metastases show sialyl transferase values of more than 74.8 mU/ml (2 SD above the normal mean) and 82% of patients that did not show any metastases after surgical tumor removal had less than 74.8 mU/ml enzyme activity (Table 1).

These results reflect a close correlation between enzyme activity and tumor size during different stages of the disease. We believe that determination of sialyl transferase is likely to be a relevant tool in the follow-up of cancer patients.

Method

In all our studies sialyl transferase activity was estimated in serum samples of cancer patients and controls, immobilized asialo-fetuin being used as the acceptor and cytidine-5′-monophospho-^{14}C-sialic acid as donor [5].

Results

At present we are concentrating on the observation of patients over a longer period of time. Our preliminary results for gastrointestinal and breast cancers are shown in Figs. 2 and 3.

At present, our observation period for gastrointestinal cancers is a little more than 6 months. The majority are being treated for colon cancer. At present 23 patients have not relapsed, 8 patients have shown deterioration of their clinical state during the period of observation, and

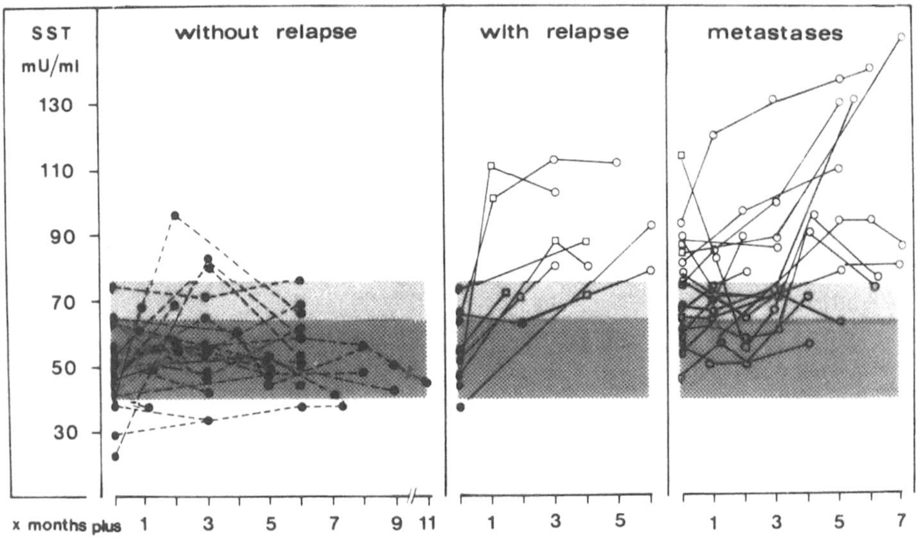

Fig. 2. Follow-up of patients with gastrointestinal cancers. The clinical state is indicated (without relapse $n = 23$, with relapse $n = 8$, proven metastases $n = 17$). - -●- -: no detectable tumor tissue: -□-: proven metastases: -○-: patients receiving chemotherapy: -□-: before surgery (primary cancer): ↓ surgical tumor removal. The dark area indicates the mean ± 1 SD for sialyl transferase activity of normal healthy subjects (50.6 ± 12.1 mU/ml), the light area the mean + 2 SD (74.8 mU/ml)

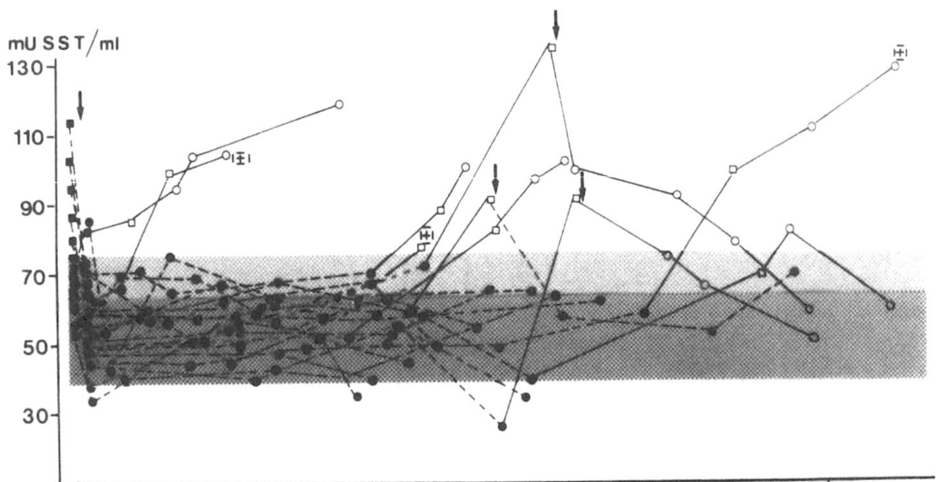

Fig. 3. Follow-up of patients with breast cancer ($n = 23$). See Fig. 2 and text for details

17 have metastases. In the case of breast cancer 23 patients are being treated and have been regularly monitored for a maximum of 3 years' observation. Eight of them have already relapsed and three patients have already died of distant metastases.

As there were no essential differences in the course of the two kinds of cancer, the clinical applicability of enzyme determination in the follow-up of malignant diseases has been

Table 2. Change of serum sialyl transferase activity with incidence of metastases compared to previous states

Without relapse	With relapse		
	< 62.7 mU/ml	62.8 – 74.8 mU/ml	> 74.8 mU/ml
< 62.7 mU/ml	0	2	6
62.8 – 74.8 mU/ml	0	0	6
< 74.8 mU/ml	0	0	1

Fifteen patients showed a deterioration in clinical state during the observation period. The change in enzyme activity is indicated above.

evaluated from combined data. So far, no correlation has been observed between the values before and after radical surgery and the incidence of metastases. Of all patients without relapse after surgery, only three with gastrointestinal tumors and one with breast cancer have shown values more than 2 SD above the mean for normal healthy subjects. At the time of examination, one patient had a benign polyp of the large-bowel mucosa, two others were suffering from temporary infection, and the last patient did not show any unusual signs. Further examination of enzyme activity indicated that this was a nonrecurring increase, as enzyme activity dropped to the initial value.

A total of 15 patients showed a deterioration of their clinical state during the period of observation, whereby metastases could be detected by X-ray, scintigraphy, endoscopy, or biopsy. The change of enzyme activity before and with the incidence of metastases is described in Table 2. Thus, 13 of 15 patients showed values above 74.8 mU/ml at the second examination, in six of whom a significant change by more than 24.2 mU/ml (more than the double SD) was seen. Only one patient showed a nonsignificant change, but even in this patient the value was more than 74.8 mU/ml. None of the cases described with relapse showed a value lower than the mean plus 1 SD (62.7 mU/ml). Thus, an increase of tumor mass was always associated with increased enzyme activity. All patients with detectable metastases were subjected to chemotherapy. Three patients with breast cancer underwent a second surgical tumor removal. There was either a local relapse of a second cancer in the corresponding mammary gland. Confirming the results of HENDERSON and co-workers, we found a close correlation between successful chemotherapy and a change in enzyme activity [8]. Therefore, serum sialyl transferase is a reliable indicator for the effectiveness of chemotherapy. If the tumor responds to treatment, a decrease in enzyme activity can be observed. In the case of ineffective treatment, enzyme activity remains at the same level or increases.

Discussion

On the basis of our results and those of other groups, we can assume that the determination of serum sialyl transferase is likely to be a relevant tool in the diagnosis and follow-up of cancer patients. It has been shown with great reliability that there is a close correlation between enzyme activity and the corresponding clinical state and that a change in the clinical course is frequently accompanied by a corresponding change in enzyme activity.

Table 3. Possible reasons for false results

False positive results
1. Infectious disease of bacterial, viral, and fungal genesis, e. g.; pneumonia, arthritis, hepatitis, herpes zoster or simplex, generalized mycoses
2. Benign tumors (proliferative mastopathies, polyps of the large-bowel mucosa)
3. Surgery 2–4 weeks before (healing process?)
4. Cell damage during therapy (e. g., adjuvant chemotherapy or radiation) and resulting from extensive tumor necroses

False negative results
1. Small primary cancers and not very extensive metastases without radiologic or scintigraphic documentation
2. Corticosteroid therapy
3. Anticoagulants (dicumarol or heparin)
4. Inappropriate sampling: Blood-clotting inhibitors (citrate, heparin, EDTA) Samples exposed to room temperature for more than 8 h, storage at −20° C for more than 2 months, heating above 40° C

Thus, serum sialyl transferase is a sensitive, but not a very specific parameter. This has been shown by possible false positive or negative results (Table 3). As all processes with enhanced cell turnover can be accompanied by enzyme activity over the normal range they can thus lead to false positive results, e.g., acute inflammation or benign tumors, following surgery and cell damage during therapy. False negative results are observed in patients with small primary cancers and not very extensive metastases without radiologic or scintigraphic proof and during medication with cortisone or anticoagulants.

In a long-term view of the field of cancer research and changed glycosyl transferases, one can speculate that at least some of these enzymes have partly tumor-associated features, e.g., isoenzymes. A first hint is the existence of the cancer-associated isoenzyme of galactosyl transferase. This was found by running serum samples in a discontinous gel electrophoretic system [11]. Until now this has not been feasible with sialyl transferase, although there are, for example, reliable differences of neuraminic acid analogues in tumor, peritumor, and normal tissue of large-bowel mucosa [12]. Only long-term clinical experience of using sialyl transferase activity as a tool in the diagnosis of malignant diseases and further biochemical findings will finally decide on its applicability.

Summary

Clinical evaluation of serum sialyl transferase as a diagnostic tool in malignant disease has shown that there is a strong correlation between enzyme activity and extent of tumor tissue. Thus, patients with large tumor masses show higher enzyme activity than patients with small tumors or in remission. Furthermore, the surgical removal of tumor tissue results in a decrease of enzyme activity to the normal range. The values remain low until metastases recur; this is connected with a new increase in enzyme activity. It has also been shown that successful chemotherapy corresponding to tumor reduction is reflected in lower values. We are thus led to believe that sialyl transferase is a relevant diagnostic blood parameter in the follow-up of cancer patients.

References

1. Bauer, Ch., Köttgen, E., Reutter, W.: Elevated activities of alpha-2 and alpha-3-fucosyl transferases in human serum as a new indicator of malignancy. Biochem. Biophys. Res. Commun. *76,* 488–494 (1977)
2. Ganzinger, U., Euler-Rolle, J., Baumgartner, G., Moser, K., Deutsch, E., Stacher, A.: Die Serum-Sialyltransferase in der Malignomdiagnostik. Verh. Dtsch. Ges. Inn. Med. *82,* 1739–1742 (1976)
3. Ganzinger, U., Dorner, F., Unger, F. M., Moser, K., Jentzsch, K.: Erhöhung der Serum-Sialyltransferase bei menschlichen Malignomen: Grundlage für ein neues Diagnosticum? Klin. Wochenschr. *55,* 553–555 (1977)
4. Ganzinger, U.: Klinische Anwendbarkeit der Serum-Sialyltransferase, Bestimmung als Maß maligne transformierter Zelloberflächenstrukturen. Wien. Klin. Wochenschr. *89,* 594–597 (1977)
5. Ganzinger, U., Moser, K., Deutsch, E.: A new diagnostic tool in human malignant disease: serum sialyltransferase. Proceedings of the 3th International Symposium on Detection and Prevention of Cancer.
6. Ganzinger, U., Baumgartner, G., Mittermayer, K., Dorner, F., Unger, F. M.: Serum-Sialyltransferase-Aktivität: Ein mögliches Hilfsmittel in der Stadieneinteilung und Verlaufskontrolle Maligner Lymphome. Verh. Dtsch. Ges. Inn. Med. *84,* (1978) (in press)
7. Ganzinger, U. et al.: (in preparation) (1978)
8. Henderson, M., Kessel, D.: Alterations in plasma sialyltransferase levels in patients with neoplastic disease. Cancer *39,* 1129–1134 (1977)
9. Kessel, D., Allen, J.: Elevated plasma sialyl transferase in the cancer patient. Cancer Res. *35,* 670–672 (1975)
10. Kim, Y. S., Perdomo, J., Whitehead, J. S.: Glycosyl transferases in human blood. I. Galactosyl transferase in human serum and erythrocyte membrane. J. Clin. Invest. *51,* 2024–2032 (1972)
11. Podolsky, K. D., Weiser, M. M.: Galactosyltransferase activity in human sera: detection of a cancer-associated isoenzyme. Biochem. Biophys. Res. Commun. *65,* 545–551 (1975)
12. Rogers, C. M., Cooke, K. B., Filipe, M. I.: The sialic acids of human large bowel mucosa: O-acetylated variants in normal and malignant states. (in press) (1978)

Evidence for Natural Antibodies (IgG) to Polyamines in Human Sera

A. M. Roch, G. A. Quash, J. P. Ripoll, and S. Saez

Introduction

It has been shown by several authors that the levels of free and/or conjugated polyamines are elevated in the urine [13], serum [1], and cerebrospinal fluid (CSF) [8] of patients with malignant diseases and with nonmalignant diseases such as cystic fibrosis [7], systemic lupus erythematosus [10], chronic infections [11], and uremia [3].
It has also been reported that when patients with malignant diseases respond to radio- or chemotherapy, serum-free polyamines (spermidine and putrescine) show an initial rise followed by a fall [9]. This fall in free putrescine and spermidine levels in CSF is well-documented for patients with neurologic tumours who have responded to treatment [8].
However, serum-free polyamines represent a fraction of the total polyamines, which, in serum, can exist in both free and bound forms [11, 12]. To try to assess the contribution of bound polyamines to this fall in polyamine levels, we began developing an inhibition of agglutination assay for bound polyamines in which human serum was used to inhibit the agglutination of latex-putrescine spheres by goat antipolyamine antiserum [2]. During development of this assay, it was observed that certain sera agglutinated latex-putrescine spheres directly. This raised the possibility that these sera contained naturally occurring antibodies to polyamines.
Qualitative evidence for these antibodies to polyamines, their specificity, and their quantitative determination in sera from normal healthy individuals and from cancer patients will be reported here.

Materials and Methods

Reagents

Carboxylated polystyrene spheres (diameter 0.3 μm) were a gift from Daniel, Rhône-Poulenc, France. N N Methylenebisacrylamide, NNN′N′ tetramethyl ethylenediamine were obtained from Eastman Kodak, Rochester N.Y., United States. Acrylamide was purchased from Fluka, Buchs, Switzerland and ammonium peroxidisulfate, Tris hydroxymethyl amino methane H_2O_2, and Tween 20 from Merck, France. Bovine serum albumin (BSA), 2-mercaptoethanol (ME), putrescine (PUT), spermidine (SPD), and spermine (SPM), the hydrochloride salts used, were purchased from Sigma Chemical Co., Saint Louis, Mo., United States. 2 2′ Azino-di-[3-ethyl-benzthiazoline sulfonate (6)] (ABTS), reference BSA, ovalbumin, and chymotrypsinogen were from Boehringer Mannheim, France. Peroxidase-labeled sheep immunoglobulins antihuman IgG γ-chain-specific were purchased from Institut Pasteur, Paris, France. Sodium dodecylsulfate (SDS) was from Sera-Feinbiochemica, Heidelberg, Germany. DEAE cellulose was purchased from Whatman Ltd., France. Coomassie Brillant Blue R was obtained from Gurr, Searle Diagnostic, Bucks, United Kingdom.

Methods

The preparation of latex-PUT spheres was carried out as previously described [2]. IgGs were isolated from human serum by ammonium sulfate precipitation and purified by chromatography on DEAE cellulose.

Reaction of Latex-PUT or Latex-Ethanolamine with Human Sera

We incubated 150 μl of human sera with 1 mg latex-PUT (20 nmol PUT/mg latex) in 2 ml buffer containing 0.2% BSA, 0.14 *M* NaCl, 0.01 *M* borate pH 8.1 (BBS) for 16 h at 37° C. For the incubation with latex-ethanolamine (20 nmol ethanolamine/mg latex), similar conditions were used. To assess inhibition by free PUT, the serum was first incubated with 5 μmol PUT for 6 h at 37° C before the addition of the latex-PUT or latex-ethanolamine spheres.

Reaction of Latex-PUT with Purified IgG

We incubated 2 mg latex-PUT (20 nmol PUT/mg latex) with 6 mg IgG in 2 ml of buffer containing 0.2% BSA, 0.14 *M* NaCl, 0.01 *M* borate-HCl at pH 8.1 for 16 h at 37° C. When inhibition assays were performed, the IgGs were first preincubated with 1 mmol SPM for 6 h at 37° C before addition of the latex-PUT spheres.

Preparation of Latex-PUT or Latex-Ethanolamine Incubated with Serum or IgG for Polyacrylamide Gel Electrophoresis

After the 16-h incubation, the latex spheres were centrifuged at 10,000 *g* for 30 min at 22°C. The supernatant was discarded and the latex pellet was resuspended in the Vortex mixer in BBS containing 0.015% Tween 20. The suspension was recentrifuged and three additional washing cycles were performed, at which point the third supernatant fluid gave no significant absorption for proteins at 280 nm. The pellet from the last centrifugation was resuspended in about 0.3 ml BBS. An aliquot of 700 μg latex was heated in a boiling water bath for 5 min with 1% SDS, 1% 2 ME, and 0.1 *M* Tris at pH 6.8.

Polyacrylamide Gel Electrophoresis (PAGE)

The treated latex (700 μg) was put on to slots in the slab gel. Preparation of the gels and electrophoretic conditions were as described by Laemmli [6]. Electrophoresis was for 16 h at 22° C with a constant current of 4 mA/gel. Gels were stained with Coomassie Brillant Blue and destained as described by Laemmli [6].

Immunoperoxidase Assay for Human IgG Bound to Latex-PUT

A 60-μg aliquot of latex washed and resuspended as described above was incubated with 50 μl of 1/50 dilution of sheep serum antihuman IgG labeled with peroxidase in 1 ml buffer containing 0.2% BSA, 0.015% Tween 20, and 0.01 *M* PO_4 at pH 7 for 1 h at 37° C and then for 16 h at 4° C. The latex spheres were centrifuged at 10,000 *g* for 30 min at 4° C. Three washing cycles with this buffer were performed as described previously. The pellet from the last centrifugation was resuspended in about 1 ml of 0.01 *M* PO_4 at pH 7 and 0.4 ml 1% ABTS and 1 ml 0.02% H_2O_2 were added. The tubes were incubated 10 min at 37° C and centrifuged at 10,000 *g* for 30 min to eliminate the latex spheres. The optical density of the supernatant was measured at 420 nm on a Zeiss spectrophotometer PMQ 3. Controls for this reaction consisted of an equivalent amount of latex spheres that had not been incubated with human sera.

Results

The inhibition of agglutination assay developed for serum polyamines involved two steps:
1. preincubation of human serum at different dilutions with the experimental goat serum at 1/5 dilution for 1 h at 37° C; and
2. addition of 100 μg latex-PUT to this mixture of sera.

When this was done it was found that the latex-PUT spheres were agglutinated to a greater extent by the serum mixture than by the experimental serum alone. There were three possible explanations for this observation:
1. Nonspecific agglutination was taking place between the latex-PUT spheres and some constituent of human serum;
2. Human serum contained antibodies to polyamines;
3. In the presence of human serum, triple complexes were formed between the antipolyamine antibodies in the experimental serum, bound polyamines in the human serum, and the latex-PUT spheres.

Qualitative Evidence for Antipolyamine Antibodies

Total Serum

To determine whether the reaction was specific, human serum was preincubated in the presence or absence of PUT before the addition of latex-ethanolamine spheres. After a further

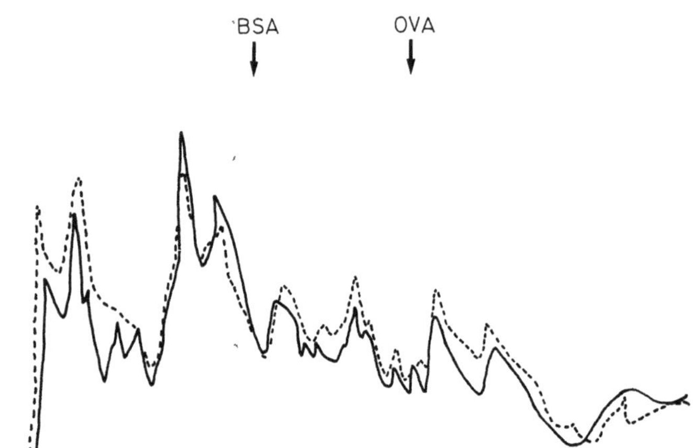

Fig. 1. Densitometer tracings of proteins obtained from latex-ethanolamine spheres incubated with human serum and separated by PAGE.
······ serum preincubated with buffer alone
——— serum preincubated with buffer containing 5 μmol PUT

incubation period of 16 h at 37° C, the latex spheres were washed by three successive cycles of centrifugation, as described earlier. Any protein adhering to the spheres was first dissociated by boiling for 5 min in the presence of 1% β-ME and 1% SDS, then separated by PAGE and stained as previously described.

Densitometer tracings of the protein bands are shown in Fig. 1, from which it can be seen that there is attachment of serum proteins that are not IgG. Further, the preincubation of the serum with PUT does not diminish the intensity of these bands. On the other hand, with latex-PUT spheres (Fig. 2), bands that correspond to the heavy (H) and light (L) chains of IgG are

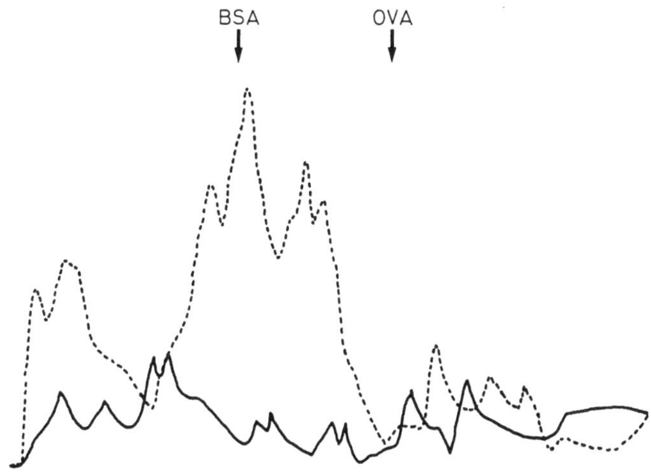

Fig. 2. Densitometer tracings of proteins obtained from latex-PUT spheres incubated with human serum and separated by PAGE.
······ serum preincubated with buffer alone
——— serum preincubated with buffer containing 5 μmol PUT

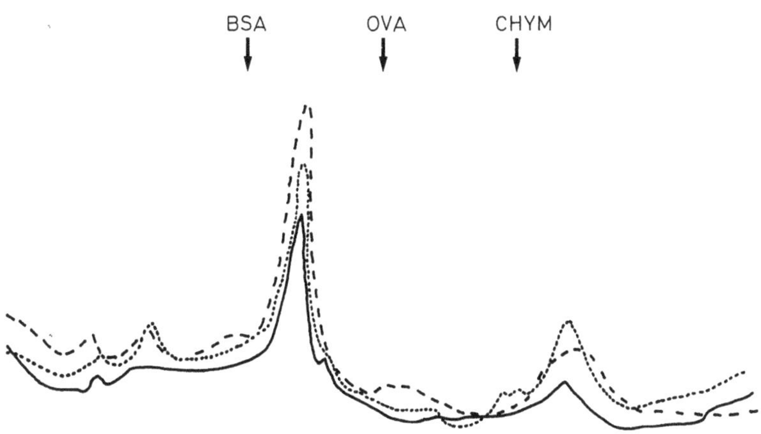

Fig. 3. Densitometer tracings of proteins separated by PAGE.
------ human IgG (control)
······ after incubation of latex-PUT with human IgG preincubated with buffer alone
——— after incubation of latex-PUT with human IgG preincubated with buffer containing 1 mmol SPM

Table 1. Inhibition of the fixation of IgG on latex-put by SPM

Origin of human IgG	Amount IgG added	BBS 0.2% BSA	BBS 0.2% BSA 1 mmol SPM	Latex for POD assay (μg)	OD at 420 nm	Inhibition (%)
Normal TK serum	6 mg	+	–	60	3.476	
		–	+	60	0.553	84
Patient 408	6 mg	+	–	60	2.650	
		–	+	60	0.796	77
Patient 409	6 mg	+	–	60	1.521	
		–	+	60	0.725	68

present and these H and L chains diminish in intensity when the serum is preincubated with PUT.

Purified IgGs

As Fig. 3 shows, IgGs purified from human sera react with latex-PUT spheres, showing two major bands corresponding to the H and L chains of IgG; the intensity of staining of these bands is reduced when the IgGs are preincubated with either PUT or SPM.

Quantitative Determination of the Amount of Antipolyamine Antibodies Reacting with Latex-PUT Spheres

Latex-PUT spheres were incubated with purified IgGs and washed as previously described. The spheres were resuspended in 0.01 *M* phosphate at pH 7 and an aliquot of this latex was reacted with a sheep serum antihuman IgG labeled with peroxidase. The results in Table 1 show that the preincubation of the IgGs with free SPM before the addition of the latex-PUT spheres inhibits the reaction by 85%.
Having obtained evidence that the serum proteins reacting with latex-PUT are IgGs and that the reaction is specific, we undertook a systematic examination of sera from cancer patients, before and after treatment, for the presence of antibodies to polyamines by the immunolatex nephelometric method previously described [4].

Discussion

The results of the polyacrylamide gel electrophoreses provide evidence for the existence of IgGs in human sera that react specifically with latex-PUT spheres and not with the latex-ethanolamine spheres used as controls. The reaction between latex-PUT and the IgGs purified from these sera can also be inhibited by free polyamines.
Further identification of the serum proteins reacting with latex-PUT as IgG has been achieved with a peroxidase-labeled antihuman γ-chain-specific serum. These three experimental ap-

proaches provide evidence for the existence of natural antibodies in human sera reacting with polyamines.

The quantitative results obtained with the peroxidase assay for human IgG from sera of normal and tumor patients suggest that the antibody titer may be less in the sera of tumor patients than in sera of normal. The immunonephelometric assay for antipolyamine antibodies presently under way should indicate whether this observation can be generalized to all sera from cancer patients or not. However, the physiologic significance of antipolyamine antibodies, bound polyamines, and free polyamines in sera will be difficult to assess until the concentrations of each of these three substances are determined on individual sera from cancer patients before and after therapy.

Summary

Human sera contain IgGs that react with latex-putrescine spheres. Identification of the IgGs has been achieved by polyacrylamide gel electrophoresis and their reaction with peroxidase-labeled antihuman γ-chain-specific antibodies. The inhibition of IgG fixation to latex-putrescine spheres by free spermine and putrescine provides evidence that these IgGs are specific for polyamines.

References

1. Bartos, D., Campbell, R. A., Bartos, F., Grettie, D. P.: Direct determination of polyamines in human serum by radioimmunoassay. Cancer Res. *35,* 2056–2060 (1975)
2. Bonnefoy-Roch, A. M., Quash, G. A.: Development of immunolatex procedures for measuring bound polyamines. In: Advances in polyamine research. Campbell, R. A., et al. (eds.), Vol. II, pp. 55–63. New York: Raven Press 1978
3. Campbell, R., Talwalkar, Y., Bartos, D., Bartos, F., Musgrave, J., Harner, M., Puri, H., Grettie, D., Dolney, A. M., Loggan, B.: Polyamines, uremia and hemodialysis. In: Advances in polyamine research. Campbell, R. A., et al. (eds.), Vol. II, pp. 319–343. New York: Raven Press 1978
4. Grange, J., Roch, A. M., Quash, G. A.: Nephelometric assay of antigens and antibodies with latex particles. J. Immunol. Methods *18,* 365–375 (1977)
5. Janne, J., Poso, H., Raina, A.: Polyamines in rapid growth and cancer. Biochim. Biophys. Acta *473,* 241–293 (1978)
6. Laemmli, U. K.: Cleavage of structural proteins during the assembly of the head of Bacteriophage T4. Nature *227,* 680–685 (1970)
7. Lundgren, D. W., Farrell, P. M., Di Sant'Agnese, P. A.: Polyamine alterations in blood of males homozygotes and heterozygotes for cystic fibrosis. Clin. Chim. Acta *67,* 357–362 (1975)
8. Marton, L. J., Heby, O., Levin, V. A., Lubich, W. P., Crafts, D. C., Wilson, C. B.: The relationship of polyamines in cerebrospinal fluid to the presence of central nervous system tumors. Cancer Res. *36,* 973–977 (1976)
9. Nishioka, K., Romsdahl, M. M., Fritsche, H. A. (Jr.), Johnston, D. A.: Polyamines in sera of patients with solid tumors. In: Advances in polyamines research. Campbell, R. A., et al. (eds.), Vol. II, pp. 265–272. New York: Raven Press 1978
10. Puri, H., Campbell, R. A., Puri, V., Harner, M. H., Talwalkar, Y. B., Musgrave, J. E., Bartos, F., Bartos, D., Loggan, B.: Serum-free polyamines in children with systemic lupus erythematosus. In: Advances in polyamines research. Campbell, R. A., et al. (eds.), Vol. II, pp. 359–367. New York: Raven Press 1978

11. Quash, G. A., Wilson, M. B.: Polyamines in human serum. W. I. Med. J. *16,* 81–91 (1967)
12. Rosenblum, M. G., Russell, D. H.: Conjugation of radiolabeled polyamines in the rat. Cancer Res. *37,* 47–51 (1977)
13. Russell, D. H., Levy, C. C., Schimpff, S. C., Hawk, I. A.: Urinary polyamines in cancer patients. Cancer Res. *31,* 1555–1558 (1971)

Dynamic and Composition of Cellular Membranes and Serum Lipids in Malignant Disorders

C. Rosenfeld, C. Jasmin, G. Mathé, and M. Inbar

Introduction

The dynamic structural organization of the surface membrane in mammalian cells is now widely accepted and in some cases even well-documented. However, the general term "membrane fluidity" commonly employed in this respect is actually complex and covers different properties of the membrane. The most prominent of these are: (a) the degree of lateral and rotational mobilities of membrane protein receptors [9, 22] and (b) the degree of viscosity of the surface membrane lipid core [6, 7, 10, 20]. These dynamic features of the cell surface membrane, which to some extent are interrelated [21], are now believed to play a major role in cellular control mechanisms that determine normal and abnormal cell growth and differentiation [2, 3, 8, 11, 15]. Moreover, since by definition, all membrane protein receptors are embedded to some extent in the membrane lipid core, the dynamic nature or the lipid domain that is determined by its lipid composition may determine to a large extent functional activities of proteins that are embedded in it.

During the last decade, with the improvement of physical techniques such as electron spin resonance and nuclear magnetic resonance, dynamic parameters of lipid layers were studied extensively, mostly with liposomes as membrane model systems. These studies have established that three main characteristics determine the physical state of a lipid region in the membrane. The most prominent of these is the molar ratio of cholesterol to phospholipids, the two major classes of lipids in mammalian cell membranes. Under physiologic conditions, with naturally occurring phospholipids and at a constant temperature, an increase in the cholesterol to phospholipid ratio will cause an increase in the rigidity of the system. The two other characteristics are the relative amount of the different phospholipids and the degree of saturation of the phospholipid acyl chains. However, recent studies in which attempts have been made to introduce these physical methods in biology have indicated that these methods are not sensitive enough for studies with intact viable mammalian cells.

With the aid of a new physical technique, based on fluorescent polarization analysis, we have recently shown that dynamic parameters of both membrane protein receptors [9] as well as membrane lipids [20] in normal and malignant mammalian cells can be analyzed on a quantitative basis. The advantage of the new method is that it is highly sensitive, accurate, and rapid, requires only a small number of cells ($1-5 \times 10^6$), and in some cases, this new method may also provide a new tool for a single cell analysis [1]. However, the most important advantage of the fluorescence polarization technique is that measurements can be carried out with normal and malignant cells under fully viable conditions. Moreover, this new method can also be employed to study dynamic parameters of serum lipids and serum lipoproteins [Glangeand and Inbar, in preparation].

Fluorescence Polarization Analysis

In recent studies we have used fluorescence polarization analysis to determine dynamic properties of artificial liposomes, isolated cellular membranes, intact cells, and serum lipids and lipoproteins. In general the new method is based on the fluorescence polarization properties of the fluorescent hydrocarbon probe 1,6-diphenyl 1,3,5-hexatriene (DPH) when embedded in the analyzed region.

For labeling of membranes or cells, a stock solution of DPH (2×10^{-3}) in tetrahydrofuran is first diluted 1000-fold with vigorously stirred buffer. Stirring is continued for 5 min at 25° C and a clear, stable aqueous dispersion of 2×10^{-6} DPH that is practically void of fluorescence is obtained [20]. One volume of the analyzed sample is then miced with one volume of the DPH dispersion and incubated at 25° C. The penetration of the DPH molecules into the membrane is witnessed by a steep increase in the fluorescence intensity of the system, which levels off after about 30 min of incubation. The labeled samples (liposomes, serum, membranes, or intact cells) are then immediately used for fluorescence polarization analysis with the aid of a special fluorescence polarization instrument (Microviscosimeter MV-1), which was developed by Elscint Ltd. in a collaborative project with our laboratory at the Weizmann Institute.

For excitation of the DPH-labeled sample, a 365-nm band generated from a 200-W mercury arc, which is passed through a polarizer, is used. The fluorescence light is then detected in two independent cross channels, equipped with polarizers after passing through a cut-off filter for wavelengths below 390 nm. Fluorescence polarization is therefore obtained by simultaneous measurements of Iv and Ih where Iv and Ih are the fluorescence intensities polarized vertical and horizontal to the direction of polarization of the excitation beam, respectively. These values relate to the degree of fluorescence polarization (P), to the fluorescence anisotropy (r), and to the total fluorescence intensity (F) by the following equations:

$$P = \frac{Iv - Ih}{Iv + Ih} \tag{1}$$

$$r = \frac{Iv - Ih}{Iv + 2\,Ih} \tag{2}$$

$$r = \frac{2P}{3 - P} \tag{3}$$

$$F = Ih(Iv/Ih + 2) \tag{4}$$

In all fluorescence measurements the temperature is controlled with a built-in solid state unit. The measurements are rapid and the microviscosimeter readout records directly the P value within less than 20 s per sample.

From the recorded P values, the actual degree of microviscosity of the system can be calculated. The treatment of this evaluation is based on the fluorescence polarization properties of a fluorophore as described by the Perrin Eq. (5) for rotational depolarization of a nonspheric fluorophore:

$$\frac{r_o}{r} = 1 + C(r)\,\frac{T \cdot \tau}{\bar{\eta}} \tag{5}$$

where r and r_0 are the measured and the limiting fluorescence anisotropies, (the limiting fluorescence anisotropy of DPH excited at 365 nm is $r = 0.362$). C is a parameter that relates to the molecular shape of the fluorophore and has a specific value for each r value, T is the absolute temperature, τ is the excited state lifetime of DPH (the excited state of DPH is $\tau = 10$ ns) and $\bar{\eta}$ is the microviscosity of the membrane domain where the DPH is embedded. As can be seen, each of the parameters of the Perrin equation can be independently and directly determined and therefore the degree of membrane microviscosity $\bar{\eta}$ can be calculated in absolute poise units.

In summary, fluorescence polarization analysis of DPH-labeled membranes, living cells, or serum can be quantitatively expressed by two different means: (a) the degree of fluorescence polarization P that is the experimental recorded unit and (b) the absolute degree of microviscosity $\bar{\eta}$. Each of these treatments is accurate since the standard deviation of the recorded P value is $\pm$ 0.005.

Dynamics of Artificial Membranes

In order to test the operational value of the method, the dynamic nature of artificial liposomes was determined. Liposomes were prepared from different phospholipids, fatty acids and phospholipids, fatty acids, and cholesterol. All liposomes were prepared by sonication, the sonicated liposomes were labeled with DPH, and the degree of fluorescence polarization (P) was determined with the microviscosimeter. From the measured P values, the degree of microviscosity ($\bar{\eta}$) was calculated. Table 1 summarizes part of these results, which indicated that three major parameters determine the dynamic behavior of a lipid domain: (a) the relative amount of the different phospholipids in the system as illustrated by the large difference between phosphatidylcholine and sphingomyelin, (b) the ratio of cholesterol to phospholipids as is shown in the comparison between phosphatidylcholine and phosphatidylcholine cholesterol liposomes, and (c) the degree of saturation of the fatty acids in the system as demonstrated by the opposite effects of the saturated fatty acid, stearic acid, as compared to the nonsaturated fatty acid, linoleic acid. The main conclusion of these experiments is that an increase in membrane microviscosity can be introduced by: (a) an increase in the relative amount of sphingomyelin in the system, (b) an increase in the ratio of cholesterol to phospholipids, and (c) an increase in the degree of saturation of the fatty acids. On the other

Table 1. Degree of fluorescence polarization and microviscosity of DPH labeled artifical liposomes of different lipid composition[a]

Lipid composition of liposomes	Fluorescence polarization	Microviscosity
Phosphatidylcholine	0.150	0.95
Sphingomyelin	0.405	18.40
Phosphatidylcholine/cholesterol (M/M)	0.306	4.64
Phosphatidylcholine + 10% stearic acid	0.240	2.38
Phosphatidylcholine/cholesterol (M/M) + 10% linoleic acid	0.067	0.32

[a] Liposomes were obtained by sonication, labeled with DPH, and all fluorescence measurements were carried out at 25° C (For preparation of liposomes, [21]).

hand, a decrease in membrane microviscosity can be obtained by: (a) an increase in the relative amount of phosphatidylcholine, (b) a decrease in the ratio of cholesterol to phospholipids, and (c) an increase in the relative amount of unsaturated fatty acids (for more details, see also ref. 7).

Dynamics and Composition of Membranes in Normal Lymphocytes and Leukemic Lymphoblasts

With the aid of the fluorescence polarization method, the dynamic nature of membrane lipids in normal lymphocytes and leukemic lymphoblasts was determined. Results summarized in Table 2 have indicated that the degree of microviscosity is high in normal lymphocytes and low in leukemic lymphoblasts. Moreover, similar results were obtained with unfractionated populations of normal lymphocytes obtained from the peripheral blood of normal donors as well as with subpopulations of normal T, B and null cells. In addition, leukemic lymphoblasts isolated from peripheral blood or bone marrow of both null-acute lymphatic leukemic (ALL) patients or from T-All show a similarly low degree of microviscosity [1, 12, 16]. Similar results were also obtained with fresh cells isolated from chronic lymphatic leukemic (CLL) patients [13] and also with lymphoblastoid cell lines established from normal and malignant origins [5].

To provide a biochemical ground to these dynamic differences between normal and leukemic lymphocytes, plasma membranes were isolated from normal and leukemic cells (Fig. 1) both from experimental animals and humans, and the lipid composition of the isolated membranes was analyzed [16, 23]. Results summarized in Table 3 have clearly indicated that the decrease in microviscosity of leukemic cells is associated with a marked decrease in the cholesterol to phospholipid ratio in the plasma membrane of the leukemic cells. Moreover, it was also found that cholesterol deficiency in acute lymphatic leukemia is greater than in chronic lymphatic

Table 2. Fluorescence polarization and microviscosity of DPH-labeled normal lymphocytes and leukemic lymphoblasts[a]

Cells	Origin	Fluorescence polarization	Microviscosity
Normal lymphocytes	Unfractionated cells (PB)	0.287	3.81
	T cells (PB)	0.285	3.73
	B cells (PB)	0.281	3.59
	Null cells (PB)	0.283	3.67
Leukemic lymphoblasts	Null-ALL (PB)	0.240	2.38
	Null-ALL (BM)	0.237	2.30
	T-ALL (PB)	0.231	2.17
	T-ALL (BM)	0.225	2.04

[a] Cells were labeled with DPH and the fluorescence measurements carried out at 25° C. ALL, acute lymphatic leukemia; PB peripheral blood cells; BM, bone marrow cells [For more details: 1, 12, 13, 16, 24].

leukemia and therefore these results are in full agreement with the microviscosity and lipid fluidity results indicating a more pronounced effect in ALL as compared to CLL. In order to provide direct experimental evidence that membrane dynamics and lipid composition are interrelated parameters, the dynamic nature of intact cells was determined as a function of lipid alteration in intact cell membranes.

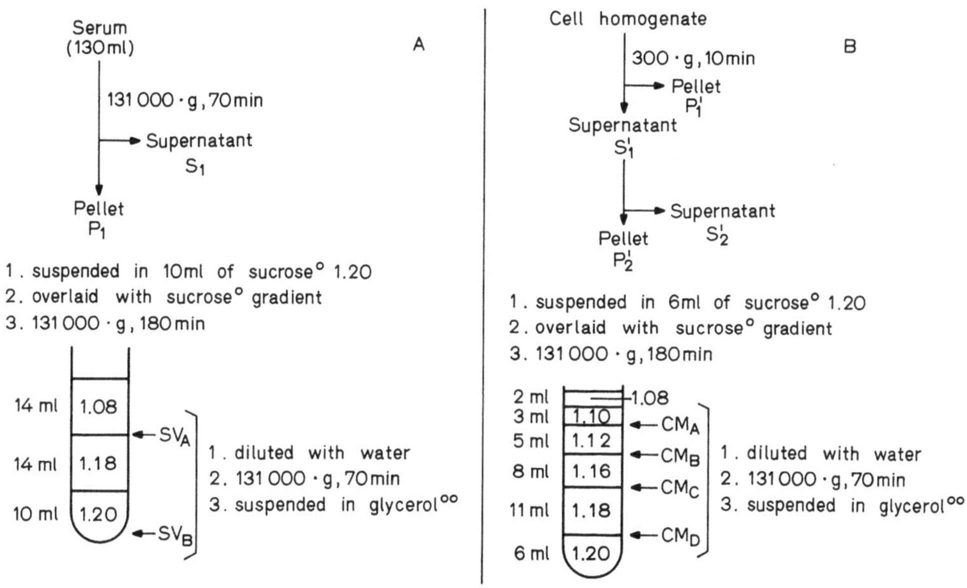

Fig. 1. Isolation and purification of membranes. **A** Serum vesicles were isolated from cell-free blood serum of leukemic patients in relapse. **B** Cellular plasma membranes were isolated from normal lymphocytes and leukemia lymphoblasts obtained from peripheral blood of normal donors and leukemic patients in relapse

Table 3. Fluorescence polarization, microviscosity, and lipid composition of plasma membranes isolated from normal lymphocytes and leukemia lymphoblasts[a]

Plasma membranes	Fluorescence polarization	Microviscosity	Cholesterol/ phospholipids (M/M)
Normal lymphocytes	0.320	5.39	0.77
	0.306	4.62	0.56
	0.320	5.39	0.74
	0.310	4.86	0.65
	0.322	5.51	0.81
Leukemic lymphoblasts	0.260	2.90	0.33
	0.275	3.37	0.41
	0.265	3.05	0.38
	0.279	3.50	0.44
	0.265	3.05	0.39

[a] For isolation of membranes and for cholesterol and phospholipids determinations: [16, 23].

Introduction of exogenous cholesterol into the surface membrane of intact leukemic cells can be performed by incubation of cells with lecithin cholesterol liposomes, and with leukemic cells such treatment resulted in an increased microviscosity and decreased lipid fluidity at a value characteristic to untreated normal lymphocytes [6, 20]. Extraction of native cholesterol from intact cell membranes can be performed by incubation of intact cells with lecithin liposomes, and therefore incubation of normal lymphocytes with lecithin liposomes resulted in a decreased microviscosity and increased lipid fluidity at a value similar to that found in untreated leukemic cells [6, 20]. The artificial changes induced in vitro in the cholesterol content and in its corresponding dynamic behavior are practically reversible for both cell types, and in principle the treated cells can assume any of these characteristics between the upper and lower limits presented by untreated normal and leukemic cells [6, 20]. These results have indeed indicated that in lymphoid cells the dynamic nature of the cell surface membrane is directly determined by the cholesterol content of the plasma membrane lipid core [16] (Tables 3 and 5).

Recently, two hypotheses have been advanced to explain the differences in cholesterol and membrane dynamics in normal and leukemic lymphocytes [16]: (a) exchange of lipids between cellular membranes and serum lipoproteins and (b) exfoliation of plasma membrane vesicles from the leukemic cell surface with a high content of cholesterol (Fig. 2).

The facile exchange in vitro of cholesterol between liposomes and intact cells of the two cell types have indicated that similar translocations of cholesterol can also occur in vivo between the cell surface membrane of lymphoid cells and blood serum lipoproteins [16]. Indeed, our results have shown that the lower level of cholesterol in the surface membrane of leukemic cell and the lower level of cholesterol in the low density lipoproteins in leukemic serum are concomitant (Table 4). Moreover, an in vitro incubation of leukemic lymphocytes with serum of isolated low density lipoproteins of normal donors results in an increased microviscosity and decreased lipid fluidity of the intact leukemic cells indicating a translocation of cholesterol from the normal serum to the leukemic cells [13, 16]. The opposite direction was observed when normal lymphocytes were incubated in leukemic serum [13, 16]. These results, part of which are summarized in Table 5, have indicated that cholesterol can be translocated from

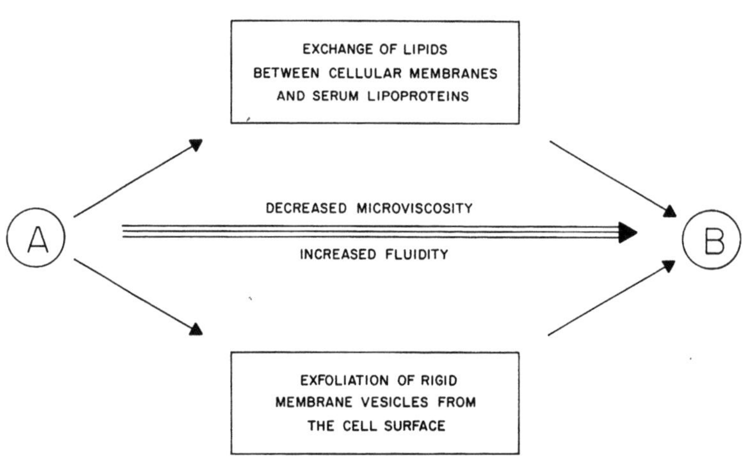

Fig. 2. Two alternative mechanisms for decreased microviscosity and increased lipid fluidity in leukemic cells

normal serum to leukemic cells and from normal lymphocytes to leukemic serum. In addition, the results have also suggested that such a translocation is specific for lymphoid cells since erythrocytes from blood of leukemic patients have the same cholesterol content as erythrocytes from normal donors [13]. The results have suggested that leukemia can be characterized by a marked reduction of cholesterol both in the plasma membrane of the leukemic cells as well as in the blood serum of the leukemic patients. It is also important to note that the rapid

Table 4. Fluorescence polarization and microviscosity of cellular membrane lipids and serum lipids in all patients in relapse and in remission[a]

Patients	Lymphocytes		Serum	
	Fluorescence polarization	Microviscosity	Fluorescence polarization	Microviscosity
ALL patients at admission or in relapse (more than 90% lymphoblasts in the circulation	0.240	2.38	0.261	2.93
ALL patients in remission for more than 20 months (less than 5% lymphoblasts in the circulation)	0.287	3.81	0.315	5.13

[a] An amount of 6×10^6 cells and 0.1 ml serum were incubated with 3 ml of DPH/PBS (2×10^{-6} *M*) for 30 min, then the fluorescence measurements were carried out at 25° C [for more details: 16].

Table 5. Changes in microviscosity of leukemic lymphoblasts induced by in vitro incubation with serum lipoproteins isolated from normal donors and by in vitro incubation with artificial liposomes of lecithin cholesterol[a]

Patient No.	Incubation for 10 h at 4° C			
	PBS	HDL	LDL	Liposomes
1	2.76	2.65	3.95	4.49
2	2.82	2.78	3.47	4.15
3	2.26	2.31	3.37	4.21
4	2.90	2.78	4.36	4.37
5	2.43	2.40	3.45	4.32
6	2.50	2.51	3.62	4.28

[a] PBS, phosphate-buffered salline; HDL, high density lipoproteins; LDL, low density lipoproteins; Liposomes, 10 mg lecithin + 5 mg cholesterol in 1 ml PBS [16].

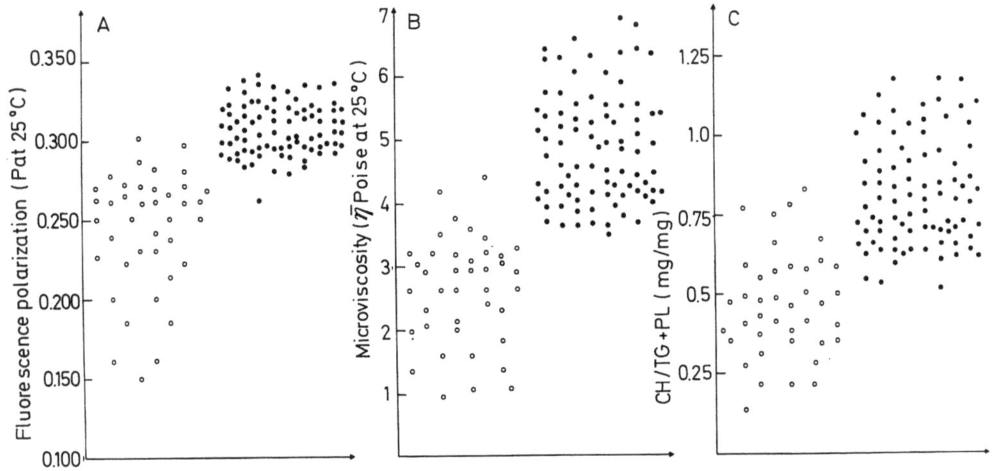

Fig. 3. Fluorescence polarization (**A**), microviscosity (**B**), and lipid composition (**C**) of serum obtained from normal donors (●) and leukemic patients (○)

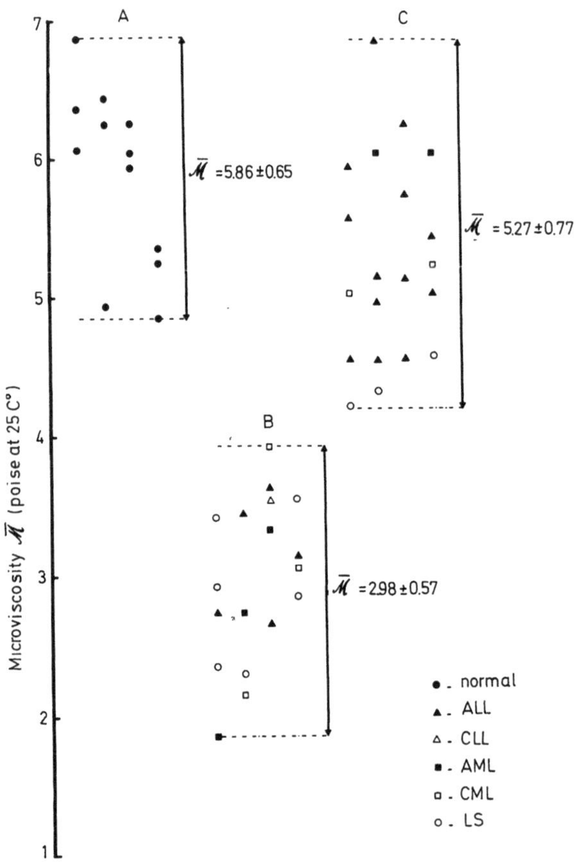

Fig. 4. Serum microviscosity. Normal donors (**A**), leukemic patients in relapse (**B**), and leukemic patients in remission (**C**)

exchange of cholesterol between leukemic cells and artificial liposomes and between leukemic cells and normal lipoproteins have indicated that leukemic cells are capable of introducing the appropriate amount of cholesterol in their membranes, once the exogenous pool of cholesterol is available [13, 16]. Moreover, a direct lipid analysis of the lipid composition of normal and leukemic serum has shown that the decreased lipid microviscosity of leukemic serum is associated with a marked decrease in the ratio of cholesterol/phospholipids and triglycerides (Fig. 3) and that the low microviscosity of serum lipids in leukemic patients in relapse increases upon remission (Fig. 4). These observations are in agreement with the notion that lipid composition and dynamics in cellular membranes of lymphoid cells and in serum lipoproteins are interrelated parameters [13, 16]. Direct evidence for this assumption was obtained from the observation that the degree of microviscosity of cells and serum decreases in leukemic patients undergoing relapse and increases in leukemic patients undergoing remission (Fig. 5).

Recent studies with mouse leukemia [17–19, 23] have shown that the development of a transplantable ascites tumor is accompanied by a significant formation of plasma membrane vesicles that can be isolated in large quantities from the cell-free ascited fluid [17–19, 23]. Similar membrane vesicles were also isolated from blood serum and pleural effusion of human leukemic patients [16] (Fig. 6). These studies have also suggested that the mechanism of vesicle formation is a specific shedding off of membrane fragments from intact viable leukemic cells [16]. A complete biochemical analysis of these vesicles has indicated that they are enriched in cholesterol. The cholesterol to phospholipid ratio in vesicles is 1 : 1, which is about threefold higher than the plasma membrane of the leukemic cells. It was concluded that their formation is one of the mechanisms whereby leukemic cells decrease their cholesterol content and therefore decrease membrane microviscosity and increase lipid fluidity (Table 6).

Our experiments have indicated that two possible mechanisms are associated with the decreased microviscosity and increased lipid fluidity of leukemic lymphocytes: (a) an abnormal exchange of lipids between leukemic cell membranes and abnormal leukemic blood serum lipoproteins and (b) exfoliation of rigid plasma membrane vesicles from the cell surface of leukemic cells (Fig. 2) [for more details: 16]. Both mechanisms are directly responsible for the low cholesterol to phospholipids ratio in the cell surface membrane of the leukemic cells.

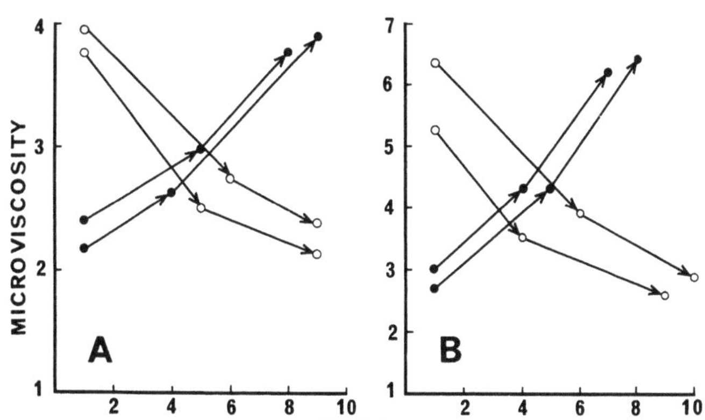

Fig. 5. Changes in microviscosity of cells (**A**) and serum (**B**) of leukemic patients undergoing remission (●) and relapse (○)

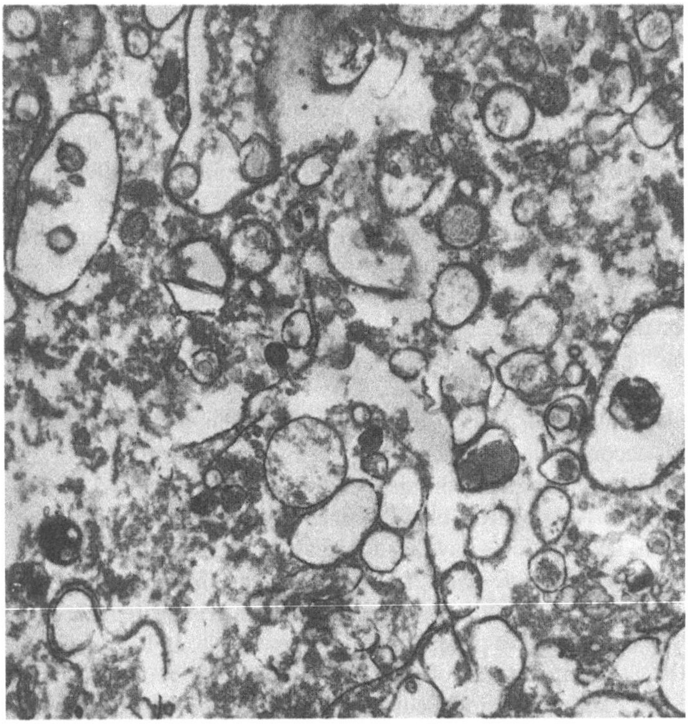

Fig. 6. Electron micrograph of membrane vesicles isolated from blood serum of leukemic patients in relapse, × 36,000

Table 6. Enzymatic activity, membrane dynamics, and lipid composition of cellular plasma membranes and serum membrane vesicles[a]

Membranes	5′-Nucleotidase (μmol Pi/mg prot/h)	Fluores. polariz. (25 °C)	Microvisco. (25 °C)	Cholesterol/ phospholipids (M/M)
Plasma membranes of normal lymphocytes	6.1	0.321	5.42	0.67
Plasma membranes of leukemic lymphoblasts	0.9	0.269	3.29	0.39
Membrane vesicles from leukemic serum	3.8	0.330	6.05	1.1

[a] For more details on the isolation of cellular plasma membranes and serum vesicles, see also Fig. 1 and [16].

Although at present there is no evidence for an interrelationship between the two mechanisms, the possibility that an abnormal exchange of lipids between cellular membranes and serum lipoproteins may have a direct effect on the degree of membrane vesiculation cannot be excluded [16].

Recent observations on mouse leukemic cells have suggested that the cell-free ascites fluid membrane vesicles also have a specific composition of membrane proteins. The specific activity of lectin receptors and of the plasma membrane enzyme marker 5′-nucleotidase was found to be higher in the vesicles than in the plasma membranes of intact leukemic cells [18, 19]. Moreover, in the YAC lymphoma, which is a Moloney virus-induced lymphoma, it was shown that the specific activity of the P-30 antigen is increased 20-fold in the membrane vesicles as compared to the YAC lymphoma cells [19]. Biologic experiments have indicated that these vesicles could be used to specifically inhibit an in vitro interaction between normal macrophages and leukemic cells [18] and that these vesicles could be used for an active immunization of mice against intact viable lymphoma cells [18, 19]. Based on these observations, it was recently suggested that the formation of such vesicles with a specific lipid and protein composition by leukemic cells may be one of the mechanisms that is responsible for the escape of leukemic cells from host immune destruction [18, 19]. In a very recent study [16] similar results were also obtained with vesicles obtained from leukemic patients in relapse (Table 6). The results have indicated that the specific activity of the plasma membrane enzyme marker 5′-nucleotidase is increased fourfold in serum vesicles as compared to isolated plasma membranes of leukemic cells (Table 6).

The two associated events that are directly related to the leukemic state, (a) the "fluidization" of cellular membranes via decrease in the ratio of cholesterol to phospholipids that may have a direct relation to increased cell proliferation and cell migration and (b) the formation of cell-free plasma membrane vesicles with a high specific activity of antigens that may have a direct relation to the increase in immunosuppression, may determine to a large extent the behavior of leukemia [16]. Based on the assumptions, an attempt was made [Yanovich, Schlossman, and Inbar, in preparation] to determine the immunogenicity of serum vesicles isolated from leukemic patients in relapse. Our results have indicated that the antiserum produced by serum vesicles have the same specificities as compared with antiserum produced by intact cells isolated from the same patient on the same day.

Some Clinical Aspects

It is evident that quantitative methods for detection of malignant or premalignant cells will prove to be of considerable value in the treatment of malignant disorders of human tissues. Therefore, one of our recent studies [14] was undertaken to determine the degree of microviscosity of lymphoid cells in ALL patients in complete hematologic remission to establish a correlation between the dynamic behavior of cellular membranes and the clinical manifestation of the disease.

Mononucleated cells isolated from 139 samples of peripheral blood obtained from 52 patients with ALL in complete hematologic remission were subjected to fluorescence polarization analysis with the aid of the fluorescent hydrocarbon probe 1,6-diphenyl 1,3,5-heatriene (DPH) when embedded in membrane lipids of intact cells. From the measured degree of fluorescence, polarization at 25° C was determined and two groups of patients were selected according to these values.

Group A included 20 patients with a mean microviscosity of 2.97 ± 0.38 and an upper limit value lower than 3.44 and group B, 23 patients with a mean microviscosity of 4.22 ± 0.38 and a lower limit value higher than 3.76. Nine patients showed an intermediate value between groups A and B. A correlation between microviscosity of cells during remission and the clinical manifestation of the disease have shown that systemic relapse, neurologic localization of leukemic cells, and death were, respectively, 2.85, 3.84, and 3.57 higher in group A than group B. These observations suggest that an abnormally low microviscosity of mononucleated cells isolated from peripheral blood of leukemic patients in complete hematologic remission, in the absence of detectable leukemic cells, may indicate an unsuccessful prognosis of the disease. Based on previous results, it was concluded that a decrease in the degree of microviscosity of a given lymphoid population is associated with an increase in the percentage of leukemic lymphoblasts. However, our recent results have shown a decrease in microviscosity of lymphoid populations without an increase in the percentage of lymphoblasts since the significant differences between groups A and B were obtained under conditions of complete absence of lymphoblasts in both groups. Moreover, none of the standard hematologic assays could distinguish between groups A and B and all 43 patients were therefore considered to be in a complete hematologic remission. The main issue of our experiments was to analyze the possibility that the low microviscosity values of patients from group A are associated with an unsuccessful prognosis as compared to patients from group B with high microviscosity values. The major idea for such a correlation stems from the observation that the microviscosity of the nonlymphoblastic populations in group A shows a leukemic-lymphoblastic behavior, whereas the microviscosity of the nonlymphoblastic populations in group B shows

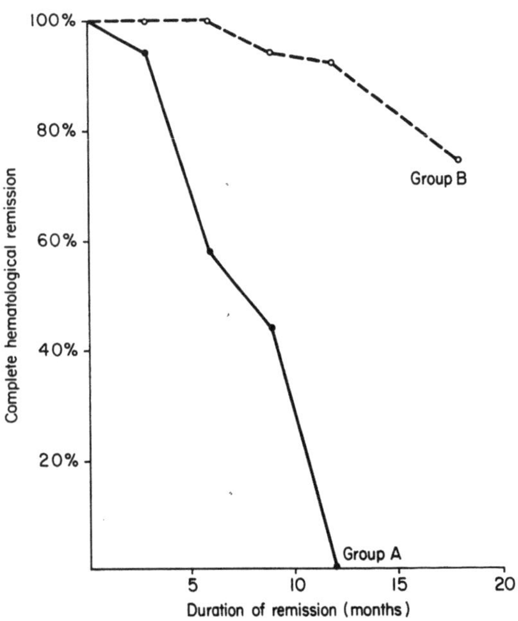

Fig. 7. Duration of remission in patients with low values of microviscosity of peripheral blood lymphocytes during remission (*group A*) and in patients with high values of microviscosity of peripheral blood lymphocytes during remission (*group B*)

normal lymphocytic behavior. For these experiments, the duration of the remission state was monitored in a selected group of 32 patients in remission both in the first or second perceptible phase. The selected group of 32 patients included 16 patients from group A and 16 patients from group B. The results summarized in Fig. 7 show that all 16 patients from group A relapsed within a period of 12 months, whereas more than 90% and 75% of the 16 patients from group B were in complete remission after 12 and 18 months, respectively. The high incidence of relapse in patients from group A suggests that low microviscosity of peripheral blood lymphocytes of ALL patients in remission may indicate for a short duration of remission and an early relapse in less than 12 months. Moreover, since the duration of remission is defined as the period of time from the induction of remission until the appearance of new lymphoblasts with low microviscosity in the circulation, it is important to note that such a characteristic can be detected months in advance of the possible detection of lymphoblasts in the peripheral blood, bone marrow, or in the central nervous system. Similar results were obtained with both null and T-ALL patients with testicular relapse [24]. Our results have shown a low degree of microviscosity of peripheral blood lymphocytes in the absence of leukemic lymphoblasts up to 6 months in advance of the detection of the testicular relapse. Based on these recent observations, microviscosity measurements are now employed as a quantitative clinical tool for early prediction of relapse in human ALL.

Concluding Remarks

The data presented in this study summarize results obtained in six different institutions throughout Europe, the United States, and Israel in the last 4 years and indicate that:

1. *Fluorescence polarization analysis with DPH* can be used for a quantitative determination of lipid dynamics both of cellular membranes and serum lipoproteins.
2. *The differences in microviscosity* between normal lymphocytes and leukemic lymphoblasts mainly originate from a difference in the ratio of cholesterol to phospholipids in the cell surface membrane of the two cell types.
3. *The decrease in the ratio of cholesterol to phospholipids* in the leukemic cells is determined by two alternative mechanisms: an abnormal exchange of lipids between the lymphoid cell membrane and serum lipoproteins and by a specific exfoliation of plasma membrane vesicles from the cell surface of leukemic cells.
4. *The two associated events* that are directly related to the leukemic state, (a) the fluidization of cellular membrane lipids via decrease in the ratio of cholesterol to phospholipids that may have a direct relation to the increase in cell proliferation and cell migration and (b) the formation of extracellular plasma membrane vesicles with a high specific activity of surface antigens that may have a direct relation to the increase in immunosuppression, may determine to a large extent the behavior of human leukemia.
5. *Microviscosity measurements of lymphoid cells* both from the peripheral blood and bone marrow and microviscosity measurements of serum lipids and lipoproteins may be clinically valuable for the early prediction of relapse.

Based on our results with leukemia, it is suggested to extend these studies to other types of malignant disorders in man.

Acknowledgement

We would like to thank the following scientists for their contributions to this project: N. Larmicol, Y. Augery, Z. Mishal, M. Petitou, F. Tuy, M. C. Glangeand, and M. Paintrand (ICIG, Villejuif); H. Ben-Bassat, A. Polliak, R. Barzilai, and G. Spira (Hadassah-Medical School, Jerusalem); P. Emmelot, W. J., Van-Blitterawijk, J. G. Collard, and J. Hilger (The Netherlands Cancer Institue, Amsterdam); B. Goldman, E. Akstein, P. Segal, and I. Ben-Bassat (Tel-Hasomer Hospital, Tel-Aviv); S. F. Schlossman and S. Yanovich (Sidney Farber Cancer Institute, Boston); A. Raz, R. Goldman, I. Bursuker, and M. Shinitzky (Weizmann Institute, Rehovot).

References

1. Ben-Bassat, H., Polliak, A., Rosenbaum, S. M., Naparstek, E., Shouval, D., Inbar, M.: Fluidity of membrane lipids and lateral mobility of concanavalin A receptors in the cell surface of normal lymphocytes and lymphocytes from patients with malignant lymphomas and leukemias. Cancer Res. *37*, 1307–1312 (1977)
2. Berke, G., Tzur, R., Inbar, M.: Changes in fluorescence polarization of a membrane probe during lymphocyte-target cell interaction. J. Immunol. *120*, 1378–1384 (1978)
3. Collard, J. G., De-Wildt, A., Oomen-Meulemans, E. P. M., Smeekens, J., Emmelot, P., Inbar, M.: Increase in fluitidy of membrane lipids in lymphocytes, fibroblasts and liver cells stimulated for growth. FEBS Lett. *77*, 173–178 (1977)
4. Inbar, M.: Fluidity of membrane lipids: A single cell analysis of mouse normal lymphocytes and malignant lymphoma cells. FEBS Lett. *67*, 180–184 (1976)
5. Inbar, M., Ben-Bassat, H.: Fluidity difference in the surface membrane lipid core of human lymphoblastoid and lymphoma cell lines. Int. J. Cancer *18*, 293–297 (1976)
6. Inbar, M., Shinitzky, M.: Cholesterol as a bioregulator in the development and inhibition of leukemia. Proc. Natl. Acad. Sci. USA *71*, 4229–4231 (1974)
7. Inbar, M., Shinitzky, M.: Increase of cholesterol level in the surface membrane of lymphoma cells and its inhibitory effect on ascites tumor development. Proc. Natl. Acad. Sci. USA *71*, 2128–2130 (1974)
8. Inbar, M., Shinitzky, M.: Decrease in microviscosity of lymphocyte surface membrane associated with stimulation induced by concanavalin A. Eur. J. Immunol. *5*, 166–170 (1975)
9. Inbar, M., Shinitzky, M., Sachs, L.: Rotational relaxation time of concanavalin A bound to the surface membrane of normal and malignant transformed cells. J. Mol. Biol. *81*, 245–253 (1973)
10. Inbar, M., Shinitzky, M., Sachs, L.: Microviscosity in the surface membrane lipid layer of intact normal lymphocytes and leukemic cells. FEBS Lett. *38*, 268–270 (1974)
11. Inbar, M., Yuli, I., Raz, A.: Contact-mediated changes in the fluidity of membrane lipids in normal and malignant transformed mammalian fibroblasts. Exp. Cell Res. *105*, 325–335 (1977)
12. Inbar, M., Larnicol, N., Jasmin, C., Mishal, Z., Augery, Y., Rosenfeld, C., Mathé, G.: A method for the quantitative detection of human acute lymphatic leukemia. Eur. J. Cancer *13*, 1231–1236 (1977)
13. Inbar, M., Goldman, R., Inbar, L., Bursuker, L., Goldman, B., Akstein, E., Segal, P., Ipp, E., Ben-Bassat, I.: Fluidity difference of membrane lipids in human normal and leukemic lymphocytes as controlled by serum components. Cancer Res. *37*, 3037–3041 (1977)
14. Larmicol, N., Jasmin, C., Augery, Y., Rosenfeld, C., Mathé, G., Inbar, M.: Prognostic values of microviscosity measurements of mononucleated cells isolated from acute lymphatic leukemia patients in remission. (submitted) (1978)

15. Levanon, A., Kohn, A., Inbar, M.: Increase in lipid fluidity of cellular membranes induced by adsorption of RNA and DNA virons. J. Virol. *22,* 353–360 (1977)
16. Petitou, M., Tuy, F., Rosenfeld, C., Mishal, Z., Paintrand, M., Jasmin, C., Mathé, G., Inbar, M.: Decreased microviscosity of membrane lipids in leukemic cells: Two possiblemechanisms. Proc. Natl. Acad. Sci. USA (in press) (1978)
17. Raz, A., Collard, J. G., Inbar, M.: Decrease in 5′-nucleotidase activity in malignant transformed and normal stimulated cells. Cancer Res. (in press) (1978)
18. Raz, A., Goldman, R., Yuli, I., Inbar, M.: Isolation of plasma membrane fragments and vesicles from ascites fluid of lymphoma-bearing mice and their possible role in the escape mechanism of tumors from host immune rejection. Cancer Immunol. Immunother. (in press) (1978)
19. Raz, A., Barzilai, R., Spira, G., Inbar, M.: Oncogenecity and immunogenicity associated with membranes isolated from cell-free ascites fluid of lymphoma-bearing mice. Cancer Res. (in press) (1978)
20. Shinitzky, M., Inbar, M.: Difference in microviscosity induced by different cholesterol levels in the surface membrane lipid layer of normal lymphocytes and malignant lymphoma cells. J. Mol. Biol. *85,* 603–615 (1974)
21. Shinitzky, M., Inbar, M.: Microviscosity parameters and protein mobility in biological membranes. Biochim. Biophys. Acta *433,* 133–149 (1976)
22. Shinitzky, M., Inbar, M., Sachs, L.: Rotational diffusion of lectins bound to the surface membrane of normal lymphocytes. FEBS Letters *34,* 247–250 (1973)
23. Van-Blitterawijk, W. J., Emmelot, P., Hilkmann, H. A. M., Oomen-Meulemans, E. P. M., Inbar, M.: Differences in lipid fluidity among isolated plasma membranes of normal and leukemic lymphocytes and membranes exfoliated from their cell surface. Biochim. Biophys. Acta *467,* 309–320 (1977)
24. Yanovich, S., Harris, K., Sallman, S. E., Schlossman, S. F., Inbar, M.: Dynamic parameters of membrane lipids in normal and leukemic human lymphocytes isolated from peripheral blood and bone marrow. (submitted) (1978)

Biologic Markers in Neuroblastoma

R. Maurus and J. Otten

Introduction

Since the introduction of adjuvant chemotherapy to the armamentarium of anticancer weapons, the question as to the optimum duration of treatment had arisen. As no marker is available for the persistence of a minimal residual tumor cell population, the chemotherapist repeatedly faces the risk of overtreating patients who are cured, or of stopping the treatment of patients who are at risk of relapse. The discovery of a sensitive and specific tumor marker should hopefully help to resolve this kind of dilemma and to improve the efficacy of the treatment. It seems paradoxical, then, that neuroblastoma, which was one of the very first cancers to be biochemically traceable, is also the malignant tumor of childhood whose prognosis has been improved only negligibly by adjuvant chemotherapy. We briefly review here some of the studies on neuroblastoma markers and the problems related to their use in everyday oncologic practice.
Table 1 presents a list of the different tests that have been used or could be used for the diagnosis and/or the follow-up of neuroblastoma.

Table 1. Biological markers in neuroblastoma

Catecholamines
Catecholamine metabolites
Dopamine β-hydroxylase
Cystathionine
CEA
Immunologic tests

Catecholamines and Catecholamine Metabolites

Neuroblastoma cells are derived from the neural crest and share with ganglioneuroma and pheochromocytoma similar biochemical properties, i.e., the synthesis, uptake, and breakdown of catecholamines. The very first reports on biochemical abnormalities in children with neuroblastoma concerned the excessive urinary excretion of noradrenalin and adrenaline, as in patients with pheochromocytoma [19, 22, 26]. Later, it was repeatedly shown that the production of adrenaline by neuroblastomas is very unusual, that noradrenalin is often only slightly increased but that dopamine or catecholamime catabolites are often excreted in high amounts by neuroblastoma patients. A simplified scheme of catecholamine synthesis and breakdown is described in Fig. 1.

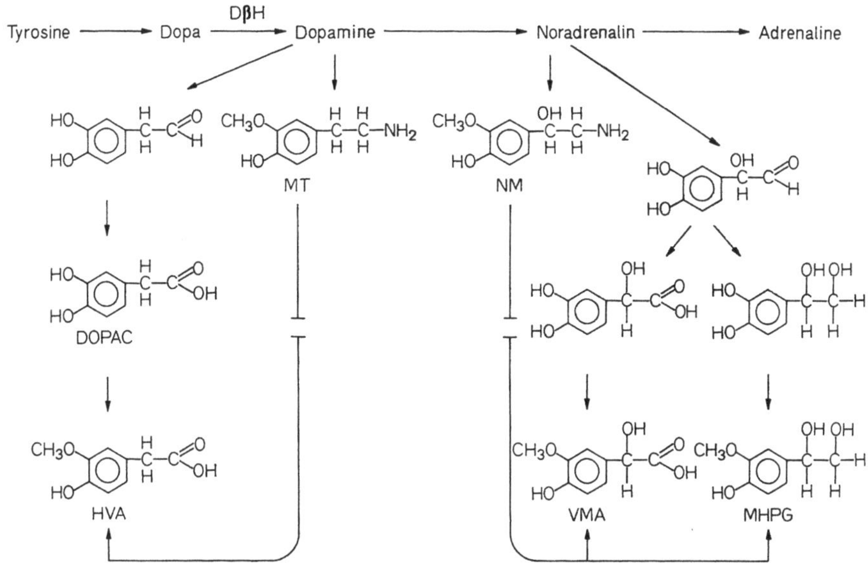

Fig. 1. Simplified scheme of catecholamine metabolism. *MT* 3-methoxy-tyramine; *NM* normetanephrine; *DOPAC* dihydroxyphenylacetic acid; *VMA* vanillylmandelic acid; *MHPG* 3-methoxy-4-hydroxy-phenylglycol

Methodology

The most commonly assayed catabolites of catecholamines are vanillylmandelic acid (VMA) and homovanillic acid (HVA). Many hospital laboratories determine only VMA by nonspecific colorimetric methods without previous purification of the metabolite. This procedure is subject to interference by many exogenous and endogenous aromatic substances. It requires the elimination of vanilla-rich foodstuffs from the diet for 3 days. If the urine is to be collected at home, any departure from the diet may give rise to false increased values.

VMA and HVA can be simultaneously determined by bidirectional paper chromatography [3]. Thin layer chromatography followed by spraying with diazotized paranitroaniline allows for rapid semiquantitative assessment of spots corresponding to several metabolites (VMA, HVA, MHPH, iso-HVA, etc.) and possibly precise colorimetric determination of each substance [8, 15, 20]. These methods require no dietary preparation of the patient.

Recently, sensitive and specific gas liquid chromatographic methods for VMA and HVA determinations have been developed, but these are unlikely to be applicable in routine clinical laboratories. Among the other metabolites, those of greatest interest are dopamine, which can be measured by various fluorimetric and gas chromatographic methods [6, 7, 16], and MHPG, for which a gas liquid chromatographic procedure has provided a sensitive assay [30].

Normal Values

Normal values as reported in the literature are expressed in different ways, in terms either of urine collection time (24 h) or of the amount of urinary creatinine. They may be established per age group, per unit of body surface area, and per unit of weight. In view of this and of the variable specificity of the multiple-assay methods used, comparison of normal values given by different authors is often difficult. VOORHESS strongly recommended 24-h urine collection on account of the great diurnal variability of catecholamine excretion [29]. However, the excretion of catecholamine catabolites, when expressed per milligram creatinine, seems much more stable than that of the catecholamines themselves, and GITLOW et al. have shown that the variation over the day is no greater than that sometimes observed between different 24-h collections in the same child [11].

As in small children, and perhaps at any age, it is difficult to avoid some urine losses, it is probably more efficient, and is certainly less inconvenient for the child, to express catabolite excretion as a function of creatinine content. The variation with age should, however, be taken into account, i.e., the gradual decrease in catabolite excretion expressed per milligram creatinine with increasing age.

The great majority of neuroblastomas can be diagnosed by the determination of VMA excretion only (Table 2). There is some discrepancy in the percentage of VMA excretors between different reported series, the reason for which is not always clear. It may be related to the lack of specificity of certain assay methods or to the unreliability of 24-h urine collections when the values are expressed as a function of time. When other metabolites such as HVA or MHPG are determined as well, positive biochemical findings are recorded in almost 100% of patients. Few authors have systematically studied dopamine excretion. KÄSER and WAGNER found this catecholamine to be increased in all their patients with neuroblastoma or ganglio-neuroblastoma [21].

It is often asserted that determination of a broader spectrum of different catecholamine metabolites makes biochemical detection of a higher percentage of neuroblastomas possible. One should, however, be cautious before accepting this diagnosis when a single poorly studied catecholamine metabolite is excreted in increased amounts. We made such a mistake in a child with a retroperitoneal extrarenal Wilm's tumor who excreted normal amounts of VMA and HVA but unusual quantities of iso-HVA (detected on thin layer chromatography). We should have been aware that some normal children may excrete detectable levels of this catabolite. The determination of metabolites other than VMA not only aids in the diagnosis but also gives some information of the prognosis. A more marked increase of HVA than of VMA is correlated with a bad prognosis.

Table 2. Percentage of neuroblastoma patients with increased excretion of catecholamine metabolites

Authors	VMA		HVA		DA		MHPG	
	%	No.	%	No.	%	No.	%	No.
Voorhess and Gardner (1962) [32]	60	17						
von Studnitz et al. (1963) [30]	96	25	68	25				
McKendrick and Edwards (1970) [27]	77	13						
Gitlow (1970) [12]	96	113	93	37			97	113
Barontini et al. (1970) [4]	87	40						
Käser and Wagner (1974) [23]	88	312	71	312	100	312		
Zücker et al. (1974) [36]	75	265	82	233	80	51		

VMA Vanillyl-mandelic acid; *HVA* Homovanillic acid; *DA* Dopamine; *MHPG* 3-methoxy-4-hydroxy-phenylglycol; *No.* Number of patients.

Biochemical Follow-up of Neuroblastoma Patients

VOORHESS and GARDNER first reported on the usefulness of serial catecholamine determination as a predictive test of the patient's progress and as a guide to further therapy [27]. GITLOW et al. presented convincing data showing that the efficacy of the treatment and the prognosis were correlated with the evolution of catecholamine excretion [13].

Among a group of 54 patients who could be followed up for at least 2 years, 86% of those whose catecholamine metabolite excretion became normal survived, whereas all those who maintained abnormal levels eventually died of their disease [13]. The return to normal may occur within days after complete excision of the tumor, or may be delayed for some weeks or months under adjuvant therapy. The persistence of elevated levels may help to decide whether or not to give a complementary treatment.

Many authors have reported on biochemical recurrences occurring before or independently of any clinical sign of relapse. In some of these cases the recurrences have been successfully treated with radiotherapy at the site of the primary tumor or with chemotherapy and have been followed by long biochemical and clinical remission. Fig. 2 illustrates one such case.

An 11-month-old boy was treated for a stage III neuroblastoma of the left adrenal with surgery, radiation therapy, and chemotherapy (vincristine + cyclophosphamide + adriamycin). Seven months later, increased VMA and dopamine excretion was observed, although no clinical sign of recurrence was detectable. A change in chemotherapy (peptichemio) was followed by biochemical normalization. The child has now been off therapy for 1 year and there is no evidence of disease $3\frac{1}{2}$ years after diagnosis.

Other anecdotal cases picked up in the literature suggest that a change or a reinforcement of therapy, introduced because of an isolated biochemical recurrence at a time when the tumor burden is still presumably small, may induce long-term remission and perhaps cure. However, no systematic study has been undertaken yet to evaluate the real impact, if any, of regular biochemical follow-up on the ultimate prognosis of neuroblastoma patients.

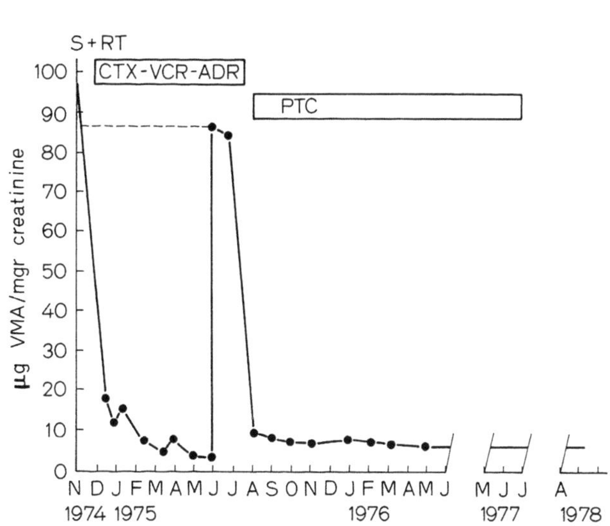

Fig. 2. Evolution of VMA excretion during and after treatment in a patient with stage III neuroblastoma

For such an evaluation, it would be appropriate to include the determination of the most sensitive markers of residual disease. In our patients, the first parameter to herald incipient relapse has usually been increased dopamine excretion. This observation was also reported by KÄSER and WAGNER [21].

There is some controversy regarding the value of bedside screening tests for the rapid semiquantitative evaluation of VMA in urine [2, 9, 24]. These methods utilize the reaction of VMA with diazotized paranitroaniline, which produces a colored product. Many other phenolic compounds interfere in this reaction, giving rise to an appreciable number of false positives. As the frequency of false negative results is also rather high (10%) [2], we think these methods too often lead to a false sense of security or to undue concern. Moreover, they screen for the presence of VMA only. As the pattern of metabolite excretion at recurrence may different from that observed at diagnosis, it may be crucial to screen for more than one substance rather than rely on VMA determination, even in patients who were VMA excretors at the initiation of treatment. Besides dopamine evaluation, we advocate the use of thin layer chromatography, which permits rapid semiquantitative estimation of VMA, HVA, MHPG, iso-HVA, etc. [8].

Other Markers in Neuroblastoma

Dopamine β-Hydroxylase (DBH)

DBH is bound to the storage vesicles in the chromaffin cells and in the postganglionic sympathetic nerve fibers and is released into the blood during exocytosis of the vesicle content. GOLDSTEIN et al. have observed an increased serum concentration of DBH in about one-half of their patients with neuroblastoma [14]. This increase was correlated with an augmented noradrenalin secretion.

Cystathionine

Cystathionine is not usually detectable in the urine of normal subjects. It has been demonstrated by column or paper chromatography in many patients with active neuroblastoma (Table 3) with or without abnormal VMA excretion [1, 10, 18]. When present, cystathioninuria disappears during remission and may herald relapse [1].

Table 3. Cystathioninuria in patients with neuroblastoma

Author	Number of patients	Percentage of patients with cystathioninuria
Geiser and Efron (1968) [10]	28	50
Helson et al. (1972) [19]	16	81
Acar et al. (1978) [1]	31	58

Carcinoembryonic Antigen (CEA)

REYNOSO et al. found elevated CEA in the serum of some children with neuroblastoma and a return to normal during remission [25].

Immunologic Reactions

Owing principally to the work by the HELLSTROMS, laboratory evidence has been accumulated to indicate the immunogenicity of human neuroblastoma cells and the presence of immunologic reactions by the host against his own tumor [5, 17]. In view of this and of the rather disappointing results of adjuvant chemotherapy in this disease, preliminary trials of combined immumo- and chemotherapy have been started in recent years. As immunotherapy may give rise to tumor enhancement, close monitoring of the immunologic reaction of the host againsts the residual disease would be mandatory. The immunologic tests described by the HELLSTROMS could form the basis of such a follow-up.

Conclusion

The great amount of information gathered over 20 years on the biochemistry of neuroblastoma has provided the clinician with reliable methods of diagnosis. They also enable him to trace clinically silent tumor cell populations and to detect incipient recurrence. Whether this last possibility has really improved ultimate control of the disease is not clearly established.

The methods used in many hospital laboratories for the evaluation of catecholamine metabolism lag far behind those developed in some research centers. It is possible that only marginal benefit is derived from the biochemical follow-up of the patients when it is restricted to the measurement of VMA excretion with rather unspecific methods. The usefulness of a frequent and detailed analysis of catecholamine metabolism in each patient remains to be evaluated.

References

1. Acar, S., Özalp, I., Büyükpamukcu, M., Tekinalp, G., Çevik, N.: The role of cystathioninuria in the diagnosis of neuroblastoma. (personal communication) (1968)
2. Addanki, S., Gombos, R. L., Hinnenkamp, E. R., Sotos, J. F.: Screening tests for vanillylmandelic acid. J. Pediatr. *90,* 955–957 (1977)
3. Armstrong, M. D., McMillan, A., Shaw, K.: 3-methoxy-4 hydroxy-D-mandelic acid, a urinary metabolite of norepinephrine. Biochem. Biophys. Acta *25,* 422–423 (1957)
4. Barontini de Gutierrez-Moyano, M., Bergada, C., Becu, L.: Catecholamine excretion in 40 children with sympathoblastoma. J. Pediatr. *77,* 239–244 (1970)
5. Bernstein, I., Hellström, I., Hellström, K. E., Wright, P. W.: Immunity to tumor antigens: potential implications in human neuroblastoma. J. Nat. Cancer Inst. *57,* 711–715 (1976)
6. Carlsson, A., Waldeck, B.: A fluorimetric method for the determination of dopamine (3-hydroxytyramine). Acta Physiol. Scand. *44,* 293–298 (1958)
7. Clarke, D. D., Wilk, S., Gitlow, S. E., Franklin, M. J.: Gas chromatographic determination of dopamine at the nanogram level. J. Gas Chromatogr. *5,* 307–310 (1967)

8. Ebinger, G., Verheyden, R., Maurus, R.: Thin-layer chromatography for diagnosis of secreting neuroblastoma. Eur. J. Pediatr. *121,* 63–69 (1975)
9. Evans, A. E.: Comment on the La Brosse VMA spot test. J. Pediatr. *86,* 240–241 (1975)
10. Geiser, C. F., Efron, M. L.: Cystathioninuria with neuroblastoma or ganglioneuroblastoma. Cancer *22,* 856–860 (1968)
11. Gitlow, S. E., Mendlowitz, M., Wilk, E. K., Wilk, S., Wolf, R. L., Bertani, L. M.: Excretion of catecholamine catabolites by normal children. J. Lab. Clin. Med. *72,* 612–620 (1968)
12. Gitlow, S. E., Bertani, L. M., Rausen, A., Gribetz, D., Dziedzic, S. W.: Diagnosis of neuroblastoma by qualitative and quantitative determination of catecholamine metabolites in urine. Cancer *25,* 1377–1383 (1970)
13. Gitlow, S. E., Dziedzic, L. B., Strauss, L.: Biochemical and histological determinants in the prognosis of neuroblastoma. Cancer *32,* 898–905 (1973)
14. Goldstein, M., Fuxe, K., Hökfelt, T.: Characterization and tissue localization of catecholamine synthesizing enzymes. Pharmacol. Rev. *24,* 293–309 (1972)
15. Gutteridge, J. M. C.: Thin-layer chromatographic techniques for the investigation of abnormal urinary catecholamine metabolite patterns. Clin. Chim. Acta *21,* 211–216 (1968)
16. Häggendal, J.: Never developments in catecholamine assay. Pharmacol. Res. *18,* 325–330 (1966)
17. Hellström, K. E., Hellström, I.: Lymphocyte-mediated cytoxicity and blocking serum activity to tumor antigens. Adv. Immunol. *18,* 209–277 (1977)
18. Helson, L., Fleisher, M., Bethune, V., Murphy, M. L., Schwartz, M. K.: Catecholamines and metabolites in patients with neuroblastoma. Clin. Chem. *18,* 613–615 (1972)
19. Isaacs, H., Medalic, M., Politzer, W. M.: Noradrenaline-secreting neuroblastoma. Br. Med. J. *1959 I,* 401–404
20. Käser, H.: Circular thin-layer chromatography for diagnosis and follow-up of neural crest tumors. J. Chromatogr. *82,* 127–136 (1973)
21. Käser, H., Wagner, H. P.: Dopamine determination for diagnosis and follow-up of neuroblastomas: experiences derived from 350 observations. Maandschr. Kindergeneesk. *42,* 449–453 (1974)
22. Mason, G. A., Hart-Mercer, J., Millar, E. J., Strang, L. B., Wynne, N. A.: Adrenaline-secreting neuroblastoma in an infant. Lancet *1957 II,* 322–325
23. McKendrick, T., Edwards, R. W. H.: The excretion of 4-hydroxy-3-methoxymandelic acid by children. Arch. Dis. Child. *40,* 418–425 (1965)
24. Ong, M., Dupont, C. L.: The La Brosse VMA spot test revisited. J. Pediatr. *86,* 238–240 (1975)
25. Reynoso, G., Chu, T. M., Holyoke, D.: Carcinoembryonic antigen in patients with different cancers. J.A.M.A. *220,* 361–365 (1972)
26. von Studnitz, W., Käser, H., Sjoerdsma, A.: Spectrum of catecholamine biochemistry in patients with neuroblastoma. N. Engl. J. Med. *269,* 232–235 (1963)
27. Voorhess, M. L., Gardner, L. I.: The value of serial catecholamine determination in children with neuroblastoma. Pedriatrics *30,* 241–246 (1962)
28. Voorhess, M. L., Gardner, L. I.: Studies of catecholamine excretion by children with neural tumors. J. Clin. Endocrinol. Metabl. *22,* 126–133 (1962)
29. Voorhess, M. L.: Discussion of: The catecholamines in tumor and urine from patients with neuroblastoma and ganglioneuroblastoma. J. Pediatr. Surg. *3,* 151–152 (1968)
30. Wilk, S., Gitlow, S. E., Clarke, D. D., Paley, D. H.: Determination of urinary 3-methoxy-4-hydroxy-phenylethyleneglycol by gas-liquid chromatography and electron capture detection. Clin. Chim. Acta *16,* 403–408 (1967)
31. Zucker, J. M.: Retrospective study of 462 cases of neuroblastoma treated between 1950 and 1970. Maandschr. Kindergeneesk. *42,* 369–385 (1974)

Immune Complexes in Breast Carcinoma

R. W. Baldwin, K. Höffken, and R. A. Robins

Introduction

Cancer-related immune complexes have been the subject of considerable interest since the demonstration that serum factors, including tumour-specific antigen-antibody complexes, could interfere with cellular immune reactivity against tumours [2, 4]. However, the microcytotoxicity test as used to measure cellular reactivity to human tumours has been the subject of considerable criticism [1, 5]. More recently, the development of sensitive and objective methods for the non-specific detection of immune complexes has allowed further investigation into the role of immune complexes in malignant disease [8]. In our laboratory, particular emphasis has been laid on the detection of immune complexes in breast carcinoma [6, 7], although similar investigations in lung cancer and osteogenic sarcoma are also in progress.

Patients and Methods

The patients in this study presented with primary operable invasive breast carcinoma and were treated by simple mastectomy. This series of patients is the subject of a wider study of determination of prognosis and response to treatment and will thus be available for long-term follow-up. Initially, immune complex levels were compared with prognosis determined by histopathological examination of lymph nodes removed at mastectomy. "Good" prognosis patients had no histological evidence of metastatic tumour in the lymph nodes, whereas "poor" prognosis patients had tumour in lymph nodes from the apex of the axilla, or internal mammary chain, or both. A "medium" prognosis group had only low axillary involvement. Plasma samples from patients and age-matched controls were tested by the modified Clq binding assay [6, 12]. Immune complexes binding ^{125}I-labelled Clq are selectively precipitated using polyethylene glycol, and results expressed as a percentage of the total Clq label precipitable with trichloracetic acid.

Results

Relationship of Plasma Clq Binding Activity to Prognosis

Plasma Clq binding activity is significantly elevated in samples taken preoperatively from breast carcinoma patients, in comparison with samples from age-matched female donors. Moreover, higher plasma Clq binding activity was found in the medium and poor prognosis patients, i.e. those with regional nodes involved with tumour, in comparison with those patients without regional lymph node involvement ("good" prognosis). When plasma sam-

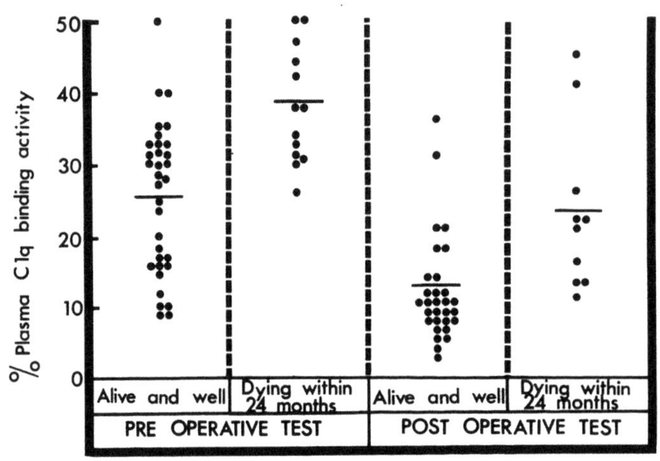

Fig. 1. Plasma Clq binding activity and 2-year survival in breast carcinoma

ples taken 12 months postmastectomy were tested, those from the good prognosis group returned to normal levels, whereas those from the medium and poor prognosis groups remained elevated.

Plasma Clq Binding and 2-Year Survival

Premastectomy and 12 months postmastectomy plasma Clq binding levels in patients dying within 2 years of mastectomy in comparison with those of patients alive and well 2 years postmastectomy are shown in Fig. 1. In the premastectomy tests, higher Clq binding values are associated with a poor clinical outcome, and 12 months postmastectomy, the Clq binding values of patients well at 2 years have generally returned to normal; postmastectomy values in patients dying within 2 years remained elevated.

Nature of Clq Binding Material

Immune complex assays are subject to interference by a variety of substances such as rheumatoid factors, DNA and endotoxin, as well as aggregated immunoglobulins. These factors have been shown not to be associated with elevated immune complex levels in cancer patients [9—11]. Immune complexes may also be present in a variety of non-malignant conditions, including infection, allergy, and rheumatoid, neurological and renal diseases, which must be considered when interpreting the results of immune complex assays. The complexes detected in cancer patients may be associated directly with the tumour, i.e. consist of tumour-related antigen-antibody complexes. This point has still to be resolved, but in comparable studies immune complexes containing tumour-specific antigen have been identified in the serum of rats bearing progressively growing tumours [3]. Furthermore, in studies on osteogenic sarcoma, it has been shown that addition of tumour cell extracts by patients' serum results in the formation of immune complexes as determined by Raji cell binding assay (Byers and Baldwin, unpublished findings). In preliminary studies, it has also been shown that addition of 3 *M* KCl extracts of breast carcinoma tissue to autologous serum increases the level of Clq binding. In both studies, the tumour specificity remains to be established but these findings are suggestive that the complexes contain tumour-related antigens. If this proves to be the case, then a specificity control could be included in the immune complex determination, distinguishing cancer-related complexes from those associated with other conditions. Furthermore, the complexes may provide a route to the isolation of tumour-related products that would be good candidates as markers for diagnosis and monitoring of malignant disease.

References

1. Baldwin, R. W.: In vitro assays of cell mediated immunity to human solid tumours: problems of quantitation, specificity and interpretation. J. Natl. Cancer Inst. *55,* 745–748 (1975)
2. Baldwin, R. W., Robins, R. A.: Factors interfering with immunological rejection of tumours. Br. Med. Bull. *32,* 118–123 (1976)
3. Bowen, J. G., Baldwin, R. W.: Isolation and characterization of tumour-specific antigen from serum of rats bearing transplanted aminoazo dye induced hepatomas. Transplantation *21,* 213–219 (1976)
4. Hellström, K. E., Hellström, I., Nepom, J. T.: Specific blocking factors – are they important? Biochim. Biophys. Acta *473,* 121–148 (1977)
5. Herberman, R. B., Oldham, R. K.: Problems associated with study of cell-mediated immunity to human tumours by microcytotoxicity assays. J. Natl. Cancer Inst. *55,* 749–754 (1975)
6. Höffken, K., Meredith, I. D., Robins, R. A., Baldwin, R. W., Davies, C. J., Blamey, R. W.: Circulating immune complexes in patients with breast cancer. Br. Med. J. *2,* 218–220 (1977)
7. Höffken, K., Meredith, I. D., Robins, R. A., Baldwin, R. W., Davies, C. J., Blamey, R. W.: Immune complexes and prognosis of human breast cancer. Lancet *1978 I,* 672–673
8. Robins, R. A., Baldwin, R. W.: Immune complexes in cancer. Cancer Immunol. Immunother. *4,* 1–3 (1978)
9. Rossen, R. D., Reisberg, M. A., Hersh, E. M., Gutterman, J. U.: The Clq binding test for soluble immune complexes: clinical correlations in patients with cancer. J. Natl. Cancer Inst. *58,* 1205–1215 (1977)
10. Samoyoa, E. A., McDuffie, F. C., Nelson, A. M., Go, V. L. W., Luthra, H. S., Brumfield, H. W.: Immunoglobulin complexes in sera of patients with malignancy. Int. J. Cancer *19,* 12–17 (1977)
11. Teshima, H., Wanebo, H., Pinský, C., Day, N. K.: Circulating immune complexes detected by ^{125}I-Clq deviation test in sera of cancer patients. J. Clin. Invest. *59,* 1134–1142 (1977)
12. Zubler, R. H., Lange, G., Lambert, P. H., Miescher, P. A.: Detection of immune complexes in unheated sera by a modified ^{125}I-Clq binding test. J. Immunol. *116,* 232–235 (1976)

Serum Leukocyte Inhibitory Factor in Cancer Patients (Serum LIF)

A. Fassas and M. Bruley-Rosset

The serum leukocyte inhibitory factor (serum LIF) assay has been devised to search in the serum of cancer patients for substances with lymphokine-like activity released in vivo. It is based on the principle that lymphokines should be released in vivo if cell-mediated immune reactions against tumor-associated antigens actually occur in tumor-bearing hosts. In fact, in vivo release of factors with macrophage migration-inhibitory factor (MIF) or LIF-like activities has been previously reported in animals [12] and in man [4, 9, 13]. COHEN et al. [4] were the first to show the presence of MIF in the serum of patients with lymphoproliferative diseases and later on MIF was also reported in patients with the Sezary syndrome [13] or posttransplantation hepatic dysfunction [10]. On the other hand, cancer sera were found to amplify the inhibition observed in direct LIF assays in various cancer patients [3, 5] and in BCG recipients [3].

The direct LIF assay, however, just like the MIF assay, is an in vitro method of lymphokine production by the patient's lymphocytes challenged by tumor antigens. Their response proves their competence and has been postulated to be an in vitro correlate of cellular immunity. The test, which is now used for the identification of specific antigens, employs the patient's nonseparated peripheral leukocytes and antigen prepared from tumor cells [1]. The reactive cell is the lymphocyte, whereas the granulocyte is the migrating cell that indicates whether LIF has been produced or not [7].

The technique used in the serum LIF assay has previously been described by one of us and was originally developed by Beaulieu at the ICIG, Villejuif [2]. It employs the patient's serum and nonseparated peripheral leukocytes of a normal donor as indicator cells. The migration is unidirectional (Fig. 1) and the migration index (MI) is calculated by dividing the migration

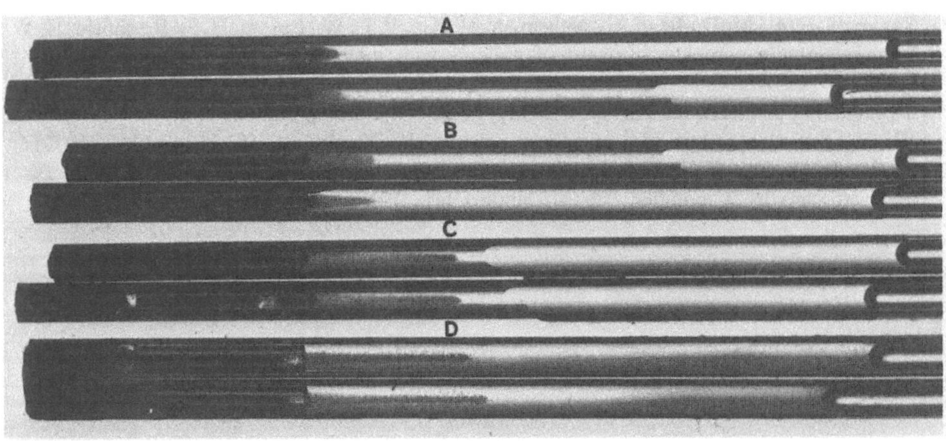

Fig. 1. Migration of normal allogeneic leukocytes in patients' sera *A and B* Migration inhibition. *C* Normal migration. *D* Control sample, i.e., leukocyte migration in normal serum

length in the patient serum by the migration length in the control (normal) allogeneic serum. Indices below 0.80 or above 1.20 are considered pathologic, indicating inhibition or enhancement.

Using this method, we have found leukocyte migration-inhibitory activity in the sera of patients with nonresectable squamous cell bronchogenic carcinoma (52/99, 53%), with metastatic breast carcinoma (13/49, 27%), with postresectional recurrent relapse of glioblastoma multiformis (21/45, 47%), with preoperative colorectal carcinoma (12/18, 67%), with acute leukemia (15/41, 37%), and with chronic myeloid leukemia in blast crisis (10/16, 63%).

Naturally, we have no clear evidence that these factors originate from lymphocytes and have anything to do with tumor immunity. However, it was interesting to find that serum LIF closely correlates with the delayed cutaneous hypersensitivity reactions to DNCB and recall antigens in the patients with the above-mentioned solid tumors (Table 1). Another interesting

Table 1. Correlation of serum LIF with cutaneous delayed hypersensitivity reactions [15]

Skin test	Skin reaction	Positive LIF tests (%)	Significance
DNCB	Positive	75 (73/97)	$P < 10^{-8}$
	Negative	14 (13/96)	
Recall antigens	Positive	88 (21/24)	$P < 10^{-9}$
	Negative	16 (8/50)	

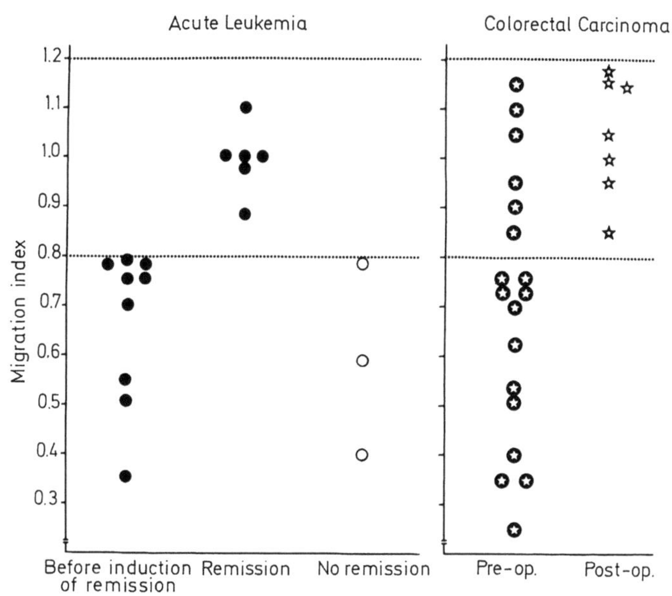

Fig. 2. Migration index values in patients with clinically detectable acute leukemia and colorectal carcinoma compared to values in the clinically nonapparent phase after treatment. Index values below 0.80 are pathologic. Sucessfully treated patients do not yield any inhibitory activity in their sera

correlation has been found with the presence of antibody in the sera of acute leukemia patients against autochtonous leukemic blasts (unpublished data), measured in cytotoxicity assays. An interesting phenomenon is also the effect of treatment on the serum inhibitory activity. As is shown in Fig. 2, patients with acute leukemia and positive sera (MI values below 0.80) do not exhibit any serum activity when they go into remission (MI values between 0.80 and 1.20), whereas if the remission-induction treatment fails to induce remission LIF can still be detected. An indirect example of the effect of treatment is shown in Fig. 2 where a group of patients with colorectal carcinoma in preoperative phase (67% positive patients) is compared to patients who have already been submitted to surgical excision of their tumor and yield normal migration results. Besides, during the maintenance chemotherapy period of acute leukemia patients, the appearance of LIF in the patient's serum seems to have a greater chance to be followed by relapse of the disease (Table 2). It appears, therefore, that serum LIF is possibly associated with the tumor and might reflect an immune reaction of the host against his neoplasm. This would necessarily suggest that immune competence is required in order to have a positive (pathologic) result, i.e., migration inhibition. If we admitted that immune competence contributes to the beneficial effect of chemotherapy, as has been postulated [6], it is not surprising to find that positive leukemic patients remit more frequently than negative ones (13/14 versus 5/10; $P < 0.06$), especially those in clinically apparent disease after their first relapse (9/10 versus 2/5; $P < 0.05$).

The difficulty lies in the interpretation of the "negative" result. This would either reflect a normal state or a state of immunosuppression. In fact, of 24 normal individuals tested, only one yielded migration-inhibitory activity in his serum [2]. Skin testing with primary or recall antigens (DHS reactions) are indispensable to discriminate between normality and immunosuppression. We tried to restore immunologically nine LIF-negative, DHS-negative patients, using BCG or poly I: poly C and, interestingly, LIF appeared in the serum of the immunorestored patients only (3/9), as determined by conversion to their DHS reactions to positive. The same thing was observed in 12 advanced cancer, anergic, and LIF-negative patients treated with chemotherapy. Five of these became reactive to recall antigens and were also converted to LIF positive. This conversion could be attributed to the decrease in tumor volume effectuated by successful chemotherapy as is also indicated by nine LIF-negative acute leukemia patients submitted to remission-induction treatment: six of these went into remission and became LIF positive, contrary to the three patients who did not remit.

One must also bear in mind the possibility that the concomitant presence of factors with opposing activities might abolish LIF in the serum as the migration enhancement factor can possibly do [11] or the chemotactic factor inhibitor that can be produced by the tumor itself [14]. The former factor is another lymphokine, considered to be secreted in vitro in cases of weak or low antigen lymphocyte sensitization [8], or in several days' lymphocyte cultures [11]. We have actually found a small proportion of migration enhancement activity in the

Table 2. Relationship of serum LIF with relapse

	Positive LIF tests (20/57)	Negative LIF tests (37/57)
Relapse	40% (8/20)	8% (3/37)
$P < 0.02$		

above-mentioned neoplastic diseases, which, interestingly, in the case of acute leukemia patients followed the same pattern of events as the inhibitory activity, disappearing after successful treatment. It seems, however, that the two factors are usually secreted separately, and if not, one is produced in excess of the other.

Preliminary results of the characterization of the serum factors showed that both the inhibitory and the enhancement activities are resistant to trypsin or pronase but may be sensitive to neuraminidase since in a number of cases they were abolished after serum treatment with neuraminidase. It seems that the terms "inhibitory factor" or "enhancement factor" include more than one factor each, and this has already been postulated for the serum MIF-like activity [13]. These serum factors also seem to be different from the factors implicated in the one- or two-step procedure migration tests employing the patient's lymphocytes.

Figure 3 shows some representative results of serum ultrafiltration on Amicon membranes and subsequent testing of the serum fractions. The inhibitory activity shown in the first three cases is contained in the low molecular weight serum fraction (< 50.000), whereas the enhancement activity that the last two cases show is contained in the high molecular weight fraction (> 50,000). Occasionally, though rarely, we find that this latter fraction also contains the inhibitory activity. The heterogeneity of the factors implicated was also seen when we separated the indicator cells by centrifuging the donor's blood in Ficoll metrizoate gradient. As far as the enhancement factor(s) is (are) concerned, it (they) seem(s) to act on the migration of granulocytes only, whereas the inhibitory activity often influences the monocyte migration as well.

In conclusion, the serum LIF assay is a more rapid and simple technique and has the advantage of detecting the in vivo release of lymphokine-like substances. Its presence in the serum possibly suggests the existence of a state of immune reactivity against tumor-asso-

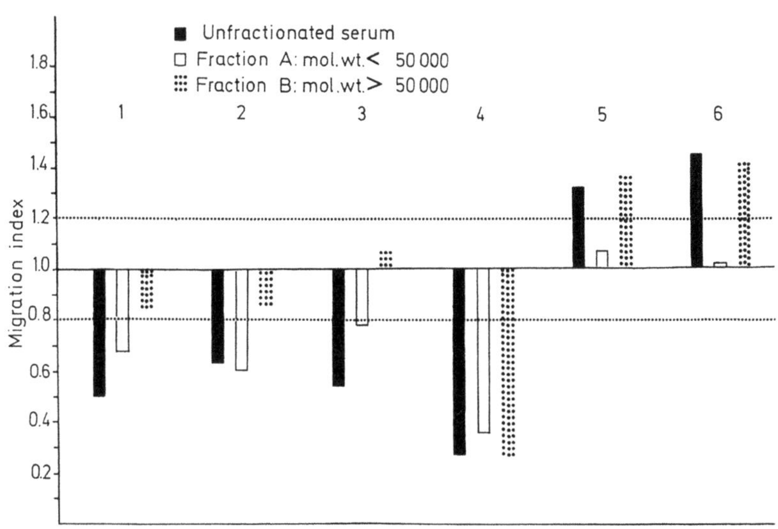

Fig. 3. Leukocyte migration in cancer sera after serum fractionation. Migration index values below 0.80 or above 1.20 are pathologic. The inhibitory activity may be contained in both serum fractions (*A* and *B*), whereas the enhancement one is always found in the high molecular weight fraction (*B*)

ciated antigens, and, as far as the clinically nonapparent phase of acute leukemia is concerned, is associated with more frequent relapse. Naturally, the patient's serum contains several substances that may or may not be related to the neoplasia, which could possibly intervene in the migration of leukocytes. Correlation of the presently described test with the direct LIF assay, which employs the patient's lymphocytes challenged by "specific" antigen, would indicate the lymphocytic origin of the serum LIF. Additionally, skin testing of the patient's immune competence should be performed simultaneously to interpret the "negative" result.

References

1. Andersen, V., Bendixen, G., Schiodt, T.: An in vitro demonstration of cellular immunity against autologous mammary carcinoma in man. Acta Med. Scand. *186,* 101–107 (1969)
2. Botto, H. G., Gauthier, H., Pouillart, P., Bruley-Rosset, M., Huguenin, P.: Correlation of delayed hypersensitivity and leukocyte migration inhibition factor in the serum of cancer patients. Europ. J. Cancer *13,* 329–332 (1977)
3. Bruley-Rosset, M., Botto, H. G., Goutner, A.: Serum migration inhibitory activity in patients with infectious dieases and various neoplasia. Eur. J. Cancer *13,* 325–328 (1977)
4. Cochran, A. J., Mackie, R. M., Ross, C. E., Ogg, L. J., Jackson, A. M.: Leukocyte migration inhibition by cancer patient's sera. Int. J. Cancer *18,* 274–281 (1976)
5. Cohen, S., Fisher, B., Yoshida, T., Bettigale, R.: Serum migration-inhibitory activity in patients with lymphoproliferative diseases. New Engl. J. Med. *290,* 882–886 (1974)
6. Lacour, F., Lacour, J., Spira, A., Bayet, S.: Effect of autologous serum on in vitro inhibition of leucocyte migration by autochtonous tumor extracts from human patients. In: Recent results in cancer research. Mathé, G., Weiner, R. (eds.), Vol. 4, pp. 129–132. Berlin, Heidelberg, New York: Springer 1974
7. Pouillart, P., Botto, H. G., Gauthier, H., Huguenin, P., Bouron, A., Laparre, C., Hoang Thy, H. T., Parrot, R., Mathé, G.: Relation entre l'état immunitaire et la réponse à la chimiothérapie. Nouv. Presse Méd. *5,* 1037–1042 (1976)
8. Rocklin, R. E.: Products of activated lymphocytes: leukocyte inhibitory factor (LIF) distinct from migration inhibitory factor (MIF). J. Immunol. *112,* 1461–1466 (1974)
9. Söborg, M.: In vitro migration of peripheral human leukocytes in cellular hypersensitivity. Acta. Med. Scand. *184,* 135–139 (1968)
10. Stastny, P., Ziff, M.: Macrophage migration inhibition and cytotoxicity in acute and chronic inflammation. In: International Congress Series No 229: Immunopathology of inflammation. Forscher, B. K., Houck, J. C. (eds.), pp. 66–73. Amsterdam: Excerpta Medica 1971
11. Torisu, M., Yoshida, T., Cohen, S.: Serum migration inhibitory activity in patients with post-transplantation hepatic dysfunction. Clin. Immunol. Immunopathol. *3,* 369–376 (1975)
12. Weisbart, R. H., Bluestone, R., Goldberg, L. S., Pearson, C. M.: Migration enhancement factor: A new lymphokine. Proc. Natl. Acad. Sci. *71,* 875–879 (1974)
13. Yoshida, T., Cohen, S.: In vivo manifestation of lymphokine and lymphokine activity. In: Mechanisms of cell-mediated immunity. McCluskey, R. T., Cohen, S, (eds.), p. 43. New York: J. Wiley 1974
14. Yoshida, T., Edelson, R., Cohen, S., Green, I.: Migration inhibitory activity in serum and cell supernatants in patients with Sezary syndrome. J. Immunol. *114,* 915–918 (1975)
15. Yoshida, T., Cohen, S.: Lymphokines in tumor immunity. In: Mechanisms of tumor immunity. Green, I., Cohen, S., McCluskey, R. T., (eds.), pp. 87–108. New York: J. Wiley 1977

Clinical Evaluation of the Modified Makari Skin Test in Minimal Residual Malignant Disease

D. E. H. Tee

Introduction

A cancer-specific antigen present in the serum of patients with carcinoma was reported by MAKARI in 1955 [5]. This antigen, antigen C, was detected by the use of the Schultz-Dale technique and was present in 96.8% of patients with carcinoma and in 4.8% with other diseases. Subsequently, MAKARI [6] reported on the presence of tumour-specific antigens that were later identified as being polysaccharidal in nature [7]. Others have confirmed the glycoprotein nature of the antigens [3, 11] and more recently, the carcinoembryonic antigens (CEA) have been demonstrated to be somewhat similar to the tumour polysaccharidal substance (TPS) described earlier by MAKARI [4].

Fairly recently, MAKARI modified the TPS antigens to enhance their sensitivity and specificity. The results obtained by a number of investigators using the modified antigens have increasingly demonstrated the value of the Makari skin test system particularly in the detection of early cancer, in the monitoring of primary treatment and in the detection of early recurrence of malignant disease after surgery [1, 2, 8–10, 12, 13]. However, its usefulness in monitoring subjects with cancer following chemotherapy and radiotherapy and its use as a prognostic indicator has yet to be defined.

The present paper describes the results of a double-blind study that was undertaken to determine the role of the modified Makari skin test in the monitoring of primary treatment and in the detection of early recurrence in patients with urological cancers.

Mechanism of Action

The mechanism by which the Makari intradermal test works in man is not fully understood, but the reaction is thought to reflect an immediate cutaneous response to complexes formed between group-specific TPSs and antibodies in the patient's serum. To prevent interference from non-tumour tisse, a tube coated with normal, inflammatory and benign tissue (NIB tube) is provided in which the patient's serum is first incubated to adsorb interfering antibodies. The test was carried out as previously described by MUNSON and TEE [9].

Monitoring Primary Treatment

Our results have shown that the diagnostic accuracy is of the order of 95% in primary untreated carcinoma, excluding anergic patients detected by means of delayed hypersensitivity skin testing [10]. A negative Makari test in an anergic patient does not exclude the presence of a tumour [1].

The results of 33 follow-up tests on patients with primary tumours have shown that eight remained positive after treatment, six of whom had residual tumour present, whilst in the other

Table 1. Results of follow-up tests on primary tumours

Initial test:	Makari positive 59			
Follow-up test:	Remaining positive 8		Converting to negative 25	
	Tumour present	Tumour absent	Tumour present	Tumour absent
	6	2	3[a]	22
Number still to be followed-up			26	

[a] Anergic – post-radiotherapy.

two there was no evidence of tumour. Of the 25 who converted to a negative reaction after primary treatment, three had tumour present. All of these had radiotherapy as their primary treatment and all were found to be anergic on repeat testing. In the remaining 22, no evidence of residual tumour was found. (Table 1).

Detection of Early Recurrence

In a group of 123 patients who had all been treated for carcinoma of the bladder and who were clinically free of recurrence, 77 gave negative and 46 gave positive results when first tested.

Table 2. Results of 48 patients followed-up for 3–9 months

Clinical follow-up	Initially negative (21)		Initially positive (27)	
	Remaining negative 13	Conversion to positive 8	Remaining positive 23	Conversion to negative 4
Recurrence-free	10	1	6[b]	4
Recurrence	3[a]	6 } 7	6 } 17	0
Positive cytology	0	1 } 7	8 } 17	0
Other primary tumour	0	0 } 7	2 } 17	0
Premalignancy	0	0 } 7	1[c] } 17	0
Concordance of test result with tumour status	10/13 (74%)	7/8 (88%)	17/23 (74%)	4/4 (100%)

[a] Anergic 3.
[b] Three patients also had intercurrent non-malignant disease (diverticular disease two, peptic ulcer one).
[c] Leukoplakia.

There were therefore 46 patients whith an unexplained positive reaction. So far 48 of these patients have been followed up, with further cystoscopic assessment and repeat Makari testing. The follow-up period ranges from 3—9 months (75 patients have not yet been followed up).

As shown in Table 2, of the 21 patients with an initial negative test, 13 remained negative, 10 are still recurrence-free, and 3 have a proven tumour but were found to be anergic on delayed hypersensitivity skin testing. Eight patients, converted from negative to positive; seven have a proven tumour (positive cytology in one), leaving one with an unexplained conversion. Of 27 patients with an initial positive test, 23 remain positive, 6 are apparently still recurrence-free, and 17 have either a suspected or proven tumour. Four patients converted from positive to negative and were recurrence-free.

Table 2 shown a high degree of concordance between the Makari test and the tumour status of the patient as determined on follow-up cystoscopy. The results contrast with those obtained initially when 46 of 123 (37%) of the patients had a positive result although apparently free of recurrence. Our current figures show that only 7 out of 48 have unexplained positive reactions, three of these have coexistent non-malignant disease. It is hoped that further follow-up will clarify the picture.

Significance

The test appears to be able to detect whether primary treatment has been adequate or not, the persistence of a positive reaction indicating that tumour is still present and conversion to a negative reaction indicating absence of tumour. However, anergic patients must be recognised, as the test result in such patients does not concur with their tumours status. The studies on "early recurrence" patients suggests that the test is capable of detecting recurrent tumour with a lead time of 3—9 months. Thus, these studies, albeit somewhat limited with regards to the number of patients and the proportion followed up so far, indicate clearly the role of the Makari skin test in minimal residual malignant diseases.

Summary

The results of a double-blind controlled study of the modified Makari skin test in urological malignancy are described. The study suggests that the test will be useful in the monitoring of primary treatment and in the detection of recurrent malignancy and thus indicates a role for the Makari skin test in minimal residual malignant disease.

Acknowledgement

I should like to thank my clinical colleagues for allowing me to study their patients, Mr. K. W. Munson, F. R. C. S., who carried out the majority of the tests and Miss Caroline Barrett for technical assistance.

References

1. Concannon, J. P., Blake, K. E., Brodmerkel, G. J., Zemel, R., Liebler, G. A., Nambisan, P. R. N.: Evaluation of the Makari Intradermal Test in the diagnosis of cancer. Ann. N.Y. Acad. Sci. *276,* 97–105 (1976)
2. Concannon, J. P., Dalbow, M. H., Eng, C. P., Blake, K. E.: Evaluation of the Makari Test for the detection of primary and recurrent cancer. Proc. 3rd Int. Detection and Prevention of Cancer (New York, April 27, 1976) New York: Marcel Dekker 1977
3. Jeanloz, R. W.: Personal communication to M. H. Goer, September 9, 1971
4. Krupey, J., Gold, P., Freedman, S. O.: Purification and characterization of carcino-embryonic antigens of the human digestive system. Nature *215,* 67–68 (1967)
5. Makari, J. G.: Use of Schultz-Dale test for detection of specific antigen in sera of patients with carcinoma. Br. Med. J. *1955 II,* 1291–1295
6. Makari, J. G.: Detection of antigens in sera of patients with neoplastic disease by Schultz-Dale test. Its possible use as a screening procedure for tumours. Br. Med. J. *1958 II,* 358–361
7. Makari, J. G.: The Polysaccharide behaviour of cancer antigens. Br. Med. J. *1958 II,* 355–358
8. Makari, J. G., Goddard, J. L.: The Makari Intradermal Test – recent studies. Proc. 3rd Int. Symp. Detection and Prevention of Cancer (New York April 27, 1976). New York: Marcel Dekker 1977
9. Munson, K. W., Tee, D. E. H.: Clinical evaluation of the Makari test in urological malignances. Br. J. Urol. *49,* 457–461 (1977)
10. Munson, K. W., Tee, D. E. H.: The modified Makari skin test in urology – is it significant? Br. J. Urol. *49,* 569–573 (1977)
11. Smith, F.: Communication to FDA. November 26, 1973
12. Tee, D. E. H.: The Makari intradermal test – recent studies. Proc. 3rd Int. Detection and Prevention of Cancer (New York, April 27, 1976) New York: Marcel Dekker 1977
13. Tee, D. E. H., Munson, K. W.: Modified Makari skin test in follow-up of bladder-cancer patients. Lancet *1977 II,* 480–481

Multiparametric Markers in the Monitoring of Cancer

E. H. Cooper

Introduction

At the present stage of knowledge about the biochemical markers in common forms of cancer, the prospects of finding specific sensitive tumour markers look bleak. Whilst the search continues, others are turning their attention to how the markers that are presently available can be used optimally [4, 8, 10].

There is a growing realisation that, with a few notable exceptions, it is unwise to depend on markers for the diagnosis of cancer or the population screening. On the other hand, the repeated measuring of markers in the same patient can provide information that relates to the evolution of disease. Furthermore, because of the complexity of cancer both in regard to the expression of tumour markers by the cancer cells and in the aberrations of biochemical homeostasis in the host, it is advantageous that more than one marker be used to follow the evolution of the disease. The confidence that an abnormal level is not a chance finding increases with the numbers of independent tests that are outside normal limits. The choice of markers to be included in a panel depends on:

a) The type of cancer to be studied, whether it has strong association with the production of a particular marker such as CEA, AFP, HCG, etc.;
b) The most likely sites of spread of this tumours, bearing in mind the impact of metastases on the levels in the blood and urine of various indicator compounds such as enzymes or the the excretion in the urine of tissue degradation products such as polyamines, β-aminoisobutyric acid and pseudouridine hydroxyproline;
c) The stage in the disease at which it is intended to use the markers and the clinical decisions that might be influenced by having appropriate intelligence about the behaviour of the cancer.

Clearly the stage of the disease can put severe restraints on markers as the levels of many of them are little affected by small loads of tumour as may be found in residual disease. A panel of markers, taken in combination with the clinical and histological staging of a primary tumour may help in assessing prognosis, even though it may only draw attention to probable understaging as is seen in large bowel cancer with subclinical metastases in the liver as indicated by a relentless rise of plasma CEA and γ-glutamyltranspeptidase levels. Clearly, a goal of such a panel would be to identify patients with micrometastases to provide more assurance that an individual patient requires adjuvant therapy other than the statistical probability that the local treatment is unlikely to have cured the disease.

A panel of markers becomes more reliable when patients are being followed after primary treatment either to monitor the onset of recurrence or to observe the effects of therapy on either localized or diffuse disease that cannot be assessed clinically, either because it is too small as in residual disease after surgery or too diffuse as in ovarian cancer.

The general logic of the selection of a tumour marker panel and the statistical examination of the results of the levels of each variate has been described by Cooper and Kenny [4].

Table 1. Main families of "markers" for monitoring cancer

Tumour-derived products
Oncofetal antigens
Carcinoembryonic antigen (CEA)
α-Fetoprotein (AFP)
Hormones
Milk proteins (casein and lactoferrin)
Methylated nucleosides, pseudouridine and β-aminoisobutyric acid
Polyamines
Enzymes and isoenzymes
Tumour-associated changes
Serum proteins – (acute phase reactants, β-2 microglobulin, immune complexes)
Pregnancy-associated proteins
Urinary hydroxyproline
Enzymes

However, as the numbers of longitudinal studies increase, it is becoming evident that the patterns of change in the levels of markers can be extremely complex and vary from one patient to another. The possibility of extraneous factors such as the alteration of the metabolism of a marker, the coincidental occurrence of two disease processes, i.e. cancer and infection, make hasty interpretation of the patterns fraught with danger. A most careful dialogue between the clinician and the laboratory is needed to identify the *cause* for the change in marker level pattern in a given patient. At best the markers can call the physicians' attention to events, but usually these tests will only be associated with a particular statistical probability that the levels of the markers will be changed by a particular event in the evolution of the cancer. In the common forms of cancer, biochemical measurement of markers is no substitute for careful clinical evaluation. Nevertheless, taken in context with the relevant clinical information they can provide an early warning of tumour progression, or the likelihood that therapy is failing to control the disease.

To catalogue all the "markers" that have been suggested is not a very helpful exercise, but it is perhaps valuable to consider some families of markers from which an appropriate selection can be made. This is presented in Table 1.

The application of the panel of marker approach can be illustrated by consideration of three types of cancer: (a) breast cancer where the oncofetal antigens provide confusing information, (b) bladder cancer that lacks good tissue specific markers and (c) the lymphomas where the classical markers have virtually no value.

Breast Cancer

The multiparametric approach to markers in breast cancer was introduced into Europe by Franchimont et al. [7]; using a panel of tumour-related antigens CEA, HCG, κ-casein, β-HCG and AFP, they found that one or more antigen was at an abnormal level in 69% at the onset of the disease (T1, T2, T3, N_0, N_1, M_0) and 88% in the presence of metastases which fell to 34% when the tumour had been removed. COOMBES et al [5] report seven tumour-index substances (acid glycoprotein, ferritin, C-reactive protein (C-RP), CEA, sialyl transferase, alkaline phosphatase and urinary hydroxyproline:creatinine ratio) were raised in 50% of 17 patients with metastatic breast cancer. However, their series was small and can be criticised for the paucity of controls. COWEN et al. [6] in a survey of 429 women attending a breast cancer clinic examined the frequency of abnormal levels of serum CEA, β-HCG, casein, γ-glutamyltranspeptidase and four acute phase reactant proteins. The profiles were unable to distinguish stages II and III from benign disease, though there was a progressive rise in the levels of the mean values of several of the parameters with increasing tumour stage, but even among the women with metastatic disease there were several in whom the battery failed to identify abnormality. C-RP was normal in 26 women without evidence of breast disease and in 55 with benign disease whilst in 3/102 (2.9%) who were clinically free of metastases after mastectomy, the C-RP was raised. However, it was only raised in 42% of stage IV cancers prior to mastectomy and this fell to 29% in metastases arising after mastectomy; this suggests it is insensitive to small tumour loads. The heterogeneity of the behaviour of the population at risk clearly emerges from COWEN's study. MACH et al. [8] summarized the situation pointing out that some markers have a limited application to specific clinical situations, such as CEA for the detection of distant metastases especially in the liver or urinary hydroxyproline: creatinine ratio for monitoring bone metastases; to this might be added serum alkaline phosphatase levels. Then there are a series of tests that may prove valuable in longitudinal studies but so far have not been studied; they include CEA, β-HCG and calcitonin levels, and the urinary production of polyamines, dimethylguanosine, pseudouridine and β-aminoisubutyric acid, the latter being of interest as it is related to t RNA [1]. After this collection of possible markers, the ground becomes very much less certain with several diverse opinions on the value of indicators such as pregnancy-associated macroglobulin, ferritin and casein.

It is apparent that in the search for early recurrence or the monitoring of the therapy of residual disease without indicator lesions relying on a single test is dangerous and illogical. The cost of providing an adequate battery may be high though it can probably be reduced once the members of the battery required for a particular patient have been identified. Unfortunately, neither of the major breast cancer adjuvant chemotherapy trials have been associated with parallel marker studies. This area of cancer research calls for a cooperative effort, and let us hope those entrusted with future trials will consider whether they might be enhanced by appropriate longitudinal studies of a panel of markers.

Bladder Cancer

Bladder cancer presents a good opportunity for the study of residual and recurrent disease as many of the forms of therapy are designed to preserve the bladder. Cystoscopic inspection, bimanual examination and when necessary biopsy are the routine clinical procedures for the surveillance against which any sets of tests need to be compared. Bladder cancer does not produce consistently abnormal levels of tumour-related antigens [10, 11], for this reason BASTABLE et al. [2] have examined whether a plasma protein profile might have some advantage in calling attention to the recurrence or the evolution of the tumour. Table 2 shows how the frequency of finding three acute phase reactant proteins with elevated levels in the serum increases with the stage of the cancer, and in particular how benign conditions and non-

Table 2. Frequency of elevation of serum three acute phase reactant proteins[a] in bladder cancer (from Bastable et al.)

	No.	Normal	One abnormality	Two or three abnormalities
T free plus controls[b]	141	131 (93%)	9 (6%)	1 (0.7%)
T1 +[c] T2 +	43	35 (81%)	7 (16%)	1 (2%)
T3 +	35	7 (20%)	6 (17%)	22 (63%)
T4 +	78	11 (14.1%)	14 (18%)	53 (68%)

[a] AGP > 1.2 g/liter; antichymotrypsin > 0.75 g/liter; C-RP > 12 mg/liter.
[b] Patients who had a cancer resected and were tumour-free. Controls = Urological patients without bladder cancer.
[c] + = Tumour present.
From Bastable et al. [2]

invasive tumours (T1) can be separated from invasive lesions. But this system cannot produce any warning about non-invasive cancer.
Longitudinal studies have shown the way the profile of acute phase reactants tents to be stable in individual patients when "in health", but the pattern becomes unstable and the levels tend to rise in response to an expanding tumour or from the tissue it is invading. Analysis of cancer-indicating substances in the urine in bladder cancer is somewhat disappointing [11]. Analysis of β-aminoisobutyric acid in the urine [12] illustrates the individual variation encountered in the excretion of this metabolite, presenting the similar type of problems as seen in breast cancer. Milford Ward et al. [9] have shown how the profile of acute phase reactant proteins can be combined with serum acid phosphatase levels to derive a discriminant function to improve the separation of prostatic cancer with and without bone metastases.

Lymphomas

This wide group of diseases often presents the problem of minimal residual disease that may readily be detected if it involved superficial lymph nodes but can often be hidden in less accessible sites. Several parameters have been suggested in the past for monitoring the lymphomas but almost characteristically they have tended to be abandoned as unreliable. In retrospect the unreliability may have been a genuine reflection of the heterogeneity of the disease. The Leeds group is assessing several possible markers in lymphomas and considers that in Hodgkin's disease (HD) and non-Hodgkin's lymphomas (NHL) a combination of serum β-2 microglobulin (β-2 m) and the C-RP levels with the ESR can provide profiles of information that draw attention to the main events in the progression [3]. The frequency of elevation of β-2 m in various forms of lymphomas is shown in Table 3. It can be seen in HD and NHL that the elevation of β-2 m is generally stage dependent. Conversely, patients in longstanding remission usually have a normal serum β-2 m. However, it is important to be certain the renal function is normal as serum β-2 m levels are elevated when the serum creatinine is $\geqslant$ 105 μM/liter [13].

Table 3. Distribution of β-2 microglobulin levels in lymphoid neoplasia

Malignant disorder	No.	β-2 m $\leqslant$ 3 mg/liter	β-2 m > 3 mg/liter
Hodgkin's disease			
Untreated			
Stages I, II	5	3	2
Stages III, IV	14	4	10
In remission < 2 years			
Stages I, II	30	29	1
Stages III, IV	12	8	4
In remission $\geqslant$ 2 years			
Stages I, II	4	4	0
Stages III, IV	7	5	2
Non-Hodgkin's lymphomas			
Untreated			
Stages I, II, E	12	8	4
Stages III, IV	32	6	26
Remission			
Stages I, II	14	13	1
Stages III, IV	17	13	4
Other Lymphoid neoplasia			
CLL	50	11	39
African Burkitt lymphoma	33	6	27
Multiple myeloma	31	4	27

A discriminant level of 3 mg/liter has been used as many of the patients tend to be in the older age group except for the Burkitt lymphomas, which were all in children, where 2.4 mg/liter would be more appropriate.

Longitudinal studies have demonstrated that whilst sometimes the elevation of β-2 m, C-RP and ESR may be highly correlated, this frequently does not occur and the time course of their changing levels produces several distinctive patterns. The simplest is seen in CLL; here the disease can be broadly divided into two groups with respect to β-2 m, though always abnormal does not rise above about 6 mg/liter, and the group whose progressive increase of β-2 m to values in the range of 10–14 mg/liter mirrors an expanding tumour load and the need for therapy, the C-RP and ESR showing relatively little change. In HD and NHL the patterns are far more complex. In certain NHL a metastable abnormal state can exist in which there may be a chronic elevation of β-2 m and ESR but with a normal C-RP, this condition can last for many months (> 20). On the other hand, the time course of levels of these indicators tends to follow the main events of the disease. Both the β-2 m and C-RP have small serum pools and short half-lives so that they can react rapidly to alterations in the patients status. The longitudinal studies have already indicated that a saw-tooth appearance of the plot of C-RP is often indicative of coincidental systemic illness, possibly of viral origin, whilst a saw-tooth behaviour of serum β-2 m levels during chemotherapy appears to be indicative of presence of residual tumour rapidly restoring the depressed β-2 m between courses. Whilst this panel of indicators can mirror many of the major events in the evolution of a lymphoma, it lacks the sensitivity needed to identify a small tumour load. As further advances in management of the lymphomas and especially NHL depends on the choice of therapy and assessment of response to therapy, future emphasis needs to be placed on the markers of tumour response. This will undoubtedly require a careful assessment of the excretion of various tumour products as well as analysis of their blood levels. The lymphomas, because of their general sensitivity, at least in the short term to therapy, would seem an ideal model to design and test a multiparametric biochemical assay of response to chemotherapy, the objective being to warn the clinician of resistance to therapy, or possibly to guide him in marking the duration and frequency of therapy making the patient's requirements.

These examples have illustrated some of the ways some contemporary markers might be used. Our experience to date suggests than non-specific biochemical changes in cancer when measured longitudinally can have a considerable information content, and they can enhance the interpretation of changes in the levels of tumour-related products should they be present.

The purpose of this brief paper is to indicate an approach to a problem and in no way to attempt to be a complete review. There are several tumours where biochemical monitoring may well be able to help clinical management. The aim of providing the physician with a biochemical warning system to use in combination with his clinical judgement seems to be attainable. However, the choice of patients needs to be considered carefully as the system is often demanding for laboratory time. Residual disease is an obvious indication for long-term study, though in the short term such studies may be used in parallel with palliative chemotherapy of larger masses to look for evidence that the patient may be deriving benefit from the therapy that is not always apparent on clinical criteria alone.

Acknowledgement

I wish to thank the clinicians who have contributed their patients to the lymphoma study and Mrs. R. Bunning, Miss S. Illingworth and Miss S. Haworth for their careful biochemical analyses. This work is supported by grants from the Yorkshire Cancer Research Campaign, The Leeds Area Health Authority with the assistance of Hoechst (United Kingdom) and Pharmacia (Sweden).

References

1. Baliga, B. S., Borek, S.: Metabolism of thymine in tumour tissue: The origins of beta-aminoisobutyric acid. Adv. Enzyme Regul. *13,* 27–36 (1975)
2. Bastable, J. R. G., Richards, B., Haworth, S., Cooper, E. H.: Acute phase reactant proteins in the clinical management of carcinoma of the bladder. (in preparation) (1978)
3. Cooper, E. H., Bunning, R., Illingworth, S., Späti, B.: Serial measurement of β2 microglobulin, acute phase reactant proteins and ESR in non-Hodgkin's lymphomas and chronic lymphocytic leukaemia. Biomedicine (in press) (1978)

4. Cooper, E. H., Kenny, T. E.: Biochemical profiles in tumour monitoring and their analysis. Proc. R. Soc. Med. *27*, 840–843 (1977)
5. Coombes, R. C., Powles, T. J., Neville, A. M.: Evaluation of biochemical markers in breast cancer. Proc. R. Soc. Med. *70*, 843–845 (1977)
6. Cowen, D. M., Searle, F., Milford Ward, A., Benson, E. A., Smiddy, F. G., Eaves, G., Cooper, E. H.: Multivariate biochemical indicators of breast cancer: an evaluation of the potential in routine practice. Eur. J. Cancer (in press) (1978)
7. Franchimont, P., Zangerle, P. F., Reuter, A., Hendrick, J. C., Molter, F.: Interest in simultaneous assays of several cancer associated antigens in various neoplastic disorders. In: Cancer related antigens. Franchimont, P. (ed.), p. 203. Amsterdam: North Holland 1976
8. Mach, J. P., Fritsche, R., Phan, M., Ozzello, L., Stjernswärd, J.: Search for biological markers in breast cancer. Prog. Clin. Biol. Res. *12*, 91–108 (1977)
9. Milford Ward, A., Houghton, A. L., Cooper, E. H.: Acute phase reactant proteins in prostate cancer. Br. J. Urol. *49*, 411–418 (1977)
10. Munro Neville, A., Cooper, E. H.: Biochemical monitoring of cancer. Ann. Clin. Biochem. *13*, 283–305 (1976)
11. Nery, P., Munro Neville, A.: Cancer indicating substances in the urine. In: Scientific foundations of urology. Williams, D. I., Chisholm, G. D. (eds.), p. 215. London: Heinemann 1976
12. Nyholm, K. K., Sjolin, K. E., Hammer, M., Knudsen, J., Stahl, D., Nielsen, H. R.: A study of the clinical significance of urinary beta-aminoisobutyric acid in patients with urothelial tumours. Biomedicine *22*, 509–516 (1975)
13. Wibell, L., Evrin, P. E., Berggard, I.: Serum $\beta 2$ microglobulin in renal disease. Nephron *10*, 320–331 (1973)

II. Adjuvant Therapies of Post-Surgical Minimal Residual Disease

A. Rational and Experimental Basis of Post-Surgical Residual Therapies

Post-Surgical Radiotherapy: Rationale and Methods

M. Tubiana

The surgeon can remove a tumor even when it is very large, but unless he performs a superradical procedure that is severely mutilating and not always effective, he often leaves microscopic disease near the line of resection.

Clinical Data

On the other hand, clinical observations and empiric knowledge founded upon experience over the last 50 years have shown that the dose required for tumor control decreases with the size of the tumor. For instance, SHUKOVSKI and FLETSCHER [31a, 12] reported that the dose that controls 90% of the squamous cell carcinomas of the supraglottic, larynx, and tonsillar fossa is 7890 rad in 8 weeks for tumors larger than 6 cm, 7300 rad in 7 weeks for tumors 4–6 cm, and 6000 rad in 6 weeks for tumors of less than 2 cm; 5000 rad in 5 weeks are sufficient for subclinical disease of the lymphatics of the neck. This decrease of the tumor control dose for small neoplastic cell aggregates is exploited in two techniques introduced 30 years ago: gradual reduction of the field size during treatment and boost.
The possibility of eradicating small cancer foci with relatively limited doses that are tolerated even when delivered on large target volumes has been used in the so-called prophylactic postoperative irradiation for over half a century. This type of adjuvant radiotherapy is widely used for tumors of the upper respiratory and digestive tract and provides good results after doses of 5000 rad in 5 weeks. For example, after surgery alone of a partial neck irradiation, the incidence of new disease in areas of the neck initially clinically negative was 11.8% (22 of 185 patients) for cancer of the nasopharynx, tonsil, and base of the tongue, whereas this incidence was only 1.7% (5 of 284 patients) when the whole neck was systematically irradiated. Similar data were reported for cancer of the floor of the mouth, oral tongue, supraglottic larynx, and pyriform sinus: 24% (46 of 187) local or regional recurrences for patients without prophylactic irradiation of clinically uninvolved neck territories versus 3% (6 of 187) for patients with prophylactic irradiation [11, 13].
Is it necessary to perform the irradiation while the disease is infraclinical? An interesting comparison was reported between two groups of patients [13]. For some, irradiation was carried out systematically immediately after surgery because there was a lack of clearance in the surgical specimen. In this group, the proportion of local control was 42%. In the other

group, radiotherapy was performed only after clinical detection of a recurrence; local control was obtained in only 11% of the patients. These results confirm that gross recurrence is more difficult to control than subclinical disease.

In breast cancer, a few randomized trials [9, 10, 45] and numerous studies [25, 39] have demonstrated that systematic irradiation with moderate doses to the thoracic wall and the axillary and supraclavicular lymph node areas significantly reduces the incidence of local and regional recurrences. For instance, when no pre- or postoperative irradiation is performed, the incidence of supraclavicular disease appearing later is 20%–25% in those patients with positive nodes in the axillary specimen, whereas when the patients are irradiated, the incidence varies between 1.3% and 7% [12]. At least 40% of the patients with T3 breast tumors without palpable lymph node have occult axillary disease; when these patients are irradiated, only about 2% develop an axillary recurrence [11, 12].

Simple mastectomy followed by postoperative irradiation obtains survival rate and recurrence-free survival equal to those observed after extended radical mastectomy [18] or radical mastectomy [17]. The effectiveness of postoperative irradiation in breast tumors is exploited in the conservative treatment of small breast tumors. After tumorectomy, irradiation of the breast and the lymph node areas is performed. For small tumors (2–3 cm), this treatment gives good cosmetic results and a survival rate that is similar to that obtained with radical mastectomy [6, 27].

For patients with soft tissue sarcomas of the extremities, local recurrences were observed in 65%–70% of the patients after surgery alone or radiotherapy alone, whereas after excision of the tumor followed by radiotherapy, the incidence was only 15% for sarcomas of the extremities and 40% for sarcomas of the head and neck and of the trunk [11].

A few studies have been performed on the clinical dose-response curve of occult residual disease. For adenocarcinomas of the breast, 3000–3500 rad control about 60%–70% of subclinical disease. For 4000 rad this proportion rises to 80%–90% and is greater than 90% for 5000 rad. for squamous cell carcinomas of the upper respiratory and digestive tract, the data are similar: 3000–4000 rad control about 60%–70% of occult residual disease and 5000 rad more than 90%. Using Cohen's mathematic model [7], Fletcher [1] calculated that 4000 rad (given in 4 weeks in 20 fractions) control 90% of aggregates containing 10^6 cells and 99% of 10^5 cell aggregates.

Similar calculations suggest that a dose of 2000 rad that is tolerated by normal tissues would cope with most tumor deposits up to about 10^5 cells. In fact, clinical experience has shown that systematic brain irradiation with doses of 2400 rad is sufficient to avoid relapses in the central nervous system during acute leukemia, and the introduction of this technique has been an important step in the curative treatment of acute leukemia.

Clinically detectable lung metastases in which there are more than 10^9 cells can hardly be controlled with radiotherapy as the dose tolerated (2000–2200 rad in 2–3 weeks) by the normal lung tissue is insufficient. However, analysis of the delay between the treatment of the primary tumor and the appearance of lung metastases suggested that in about one-third of the patients with osteosarcoma subvisual metastases have less than 10^5–10^6 cells at the time of initial treatment. This analysis provided the theoretical basis for a prophylactic irradiation of the lung in the treatment of osteosarcoma of the limb [1, 5]; a controlled clinical trial initiated in 1970 by the EORTC Radiotherapy Group confirmed that this technique significantly decreased the percentage of patients in whom metastases develop [5]. The data suggest that the occult metastases with diameters larger than a few millimeters that become visible within a few months are radioresistant, whereas the ones smaller than a few millimeters are radiosensitive [5].

Experimental Data

The results of animal studies correlate satisfactorily with the clinical data. For instance, for Lewis lung carcinoma, Shipley et al. [29] have measured the survival of the clonogenic tumor cells after in vivo irradiation. The cell radiosensitivity is much greater in a small tumor than in a large tumor. Anoxia is the main factor of radioresistance, and this difference in radiosensitivity is probably mostly due to a rapid increase of the hypoxic fraction in experimental tumors when the diameters reach 1–3 mm as suggested by the available data on tumors that have been studied (Table 1).

This observation is important not only for radiotherapy but also for chemotherapy because better tumor microvasculature also improves drug delivery and can explain the good results of systemic chemotherapy on micrometastases [32]. In this connection, it should also be noted that the amount of drug necessary for the control of experimental tumors increases very rapidly with their size [33]. However, beside hypoxia, other factors may also contribute to an explanation of the high radiosensitivity of small tumors. The mean lethal dose (D_0) of a well-oxygenated suspension of single cells originating from a tumor of 500 mm^3 and irradiated in vitro is 110 rad; it is only 89 rad for cells originating from a tumor of 0.5 mm^3 [29]. The difference, although small, is significant and might be explained by differences in cell kinetics. We have been able to demonstrate a decrease of the growth fraction during the growth of experimental tumors [15], which has subsequently been confirmed. The age-density distribution is, therefore, different in small and large tumors. Furthermore, the repair of potentially lethal damage is larger for quiescent cells, and we have shown on NCTC fibrosarcoma that the amount of repair is greater for large than for small tumors [21]. This has been recently confirmed for another type of experimental tumor, the EMT6 tumor [43].

Table 1

Type of tumor	Size of tumor	Hypoxic fraction	Ref.
C3H mammary carcinoma	0.6 mm^3 250 mm^3	0.001 0.15	Suit and Maeda [28]
EMT6 tumor	Diam. 0.5–2 mm 1 g	very low 0.3	Fu et al. [14]
Lewis lung carcinoma	0.5 mm^3 500 mm^3	0.005 0.36	Shipley et al. [29]

Criticism Against Prophylactic Irradiation

Some criticism has been raised against the use of prophylactic postoperative irradiation. The first is that it may delay systemic therapy, which is more useful because the prognosis depends on the occurrence of metastases and is not seriously influenced by regional recurrence. This is highly debatable. A survey has shown that about one-third of cancer patients die of local or regional recurrence [37], and radiotherapy is still the most effective method of preventing it.

Another criticism of the treatment of subclinical disease by prophylactic irradiation is that the presence of radiation-inactivated tumor cells results in growth of tumors with fewer viable tumor cells than without these feeder cells. This is the so-called Revesz effect. Some authors such as SCHABEL [28] have said: "curative radiation therapy in individual tumor foci may be more difficult than with surgical removal when viable tumor cells are left in situ." However, extensive surgery (e.g., radical neck dissection) is a mutilating and not always effective procedure. Secondly, it should be stressed that drug-inactivated tumor cells are as effective as irradiated cells for enhancing the growth of the surviving cells. The most important answer is that this purely theoretical assumption is not substantiated by clinical data. The reduction in the incidence of local recurrence by postoperative radiotherapy is not debated even by the critics of postoperative radiotherapy. Their reasoning is based on STJERNSWÄRD's thesis that local postoperative radiotherapy causes an increased mortality in breast cancer patients and that this harmfulness is due to an immunosuppression produced by irradiation, which enhances the incidence of distant metastases. Let us consider these two claims.

STJERNSWÄRD [36] carried out a combined analysis of the 5-year survival data from five clinical trials, temporally and geographically distinct, in which patients underwent surgery for cancer of the breast with or without postoperative irradiation. In none of these trials was significant difference between the two groups observed, but STJERNSWÄRD claimed that by pooling the results of the five trials he achieved a statistical synthesis demonstrating a significant decrease in the survival rate for the group treated by postoperative radiotherapy. However, a few authors, in particular LEVITT et al. [20], have refuted this conclusion after a careful reanalysis of the data and on the basis of statistical inaccuracies and methodologic errors.

Other data have been quoted by STJERNSWÄRD to substantiate the harmfulness of radiation. However, great caution is required in comparing series of patients who have not been randomized. There is a general tendency, conscious or unconscious, to select for postoperative irradiation those patients with the poorest prognostic indicators and in particular those for whom the surgical excision has been the most difficult or the least satisfactory. This explains why the survival rate is often higher in the unirradiated group. For instance, at Villejuif, the survival rate of unirradiated differentiated thyroid cancers is 92% at 5 years and 83% at 10 years, whereas in the group having received prophylactic postoperative radiotherapy, they are 88% and 75%, respectively [42]. This does not mean, however, that radiotherapy is harmful; on the contrary, the results obtained with high doses of telecobalt are better than those observed after moderate doses of conventional radiotherapy, which suggests the effectiveness of irradiation [41].

The depression of immunologic defenses after regional irradiation has been considered by STJERNSWÄRD et al. [35] as a serious drawback for prophylactic irradiation. First, it should be reiterated that all treatments, whether chemotherapy, extensive surgery, or even immunotherapy, are, or could be, immunodepressive in some animal systems. Secondly, it is true that a decrease in blood lymphocyte count is observed following radiotherapy, and we have been the first, to our knowledge, to report it [2]. This has been subsequently studied in a few papers [16, 24a, 35]. However, the degree of host immune competence may not necessarily parallel the number of blood lymphocytes and an induced modification of lymphocyte activity might be compensated by an immune mechanism [24b].

STJERNSWÄRD et al. [35] stated that radiation-induced lymphopenia is due to a decrease in T cells. In contrast, BLOMGREN et al. [4] observed that T cell population increased while B cell population decreased after postoperative radiotherapy of breast or bladder cancers. The least one can say is that STJERNSWÄRD's data do not substantiate his claim that local radiotherapy impairs the immune response against cancer cells [3, 20, 45]. On the other hand, cytotoxic immunity has been demonstrated following injection of radiation-inactivated homologous tumor cells with several experimental tumors, and in this situation cells killed by radiotherapy enhance the immunologic defenses [28]. For example, CRILE and DEODHAR [8] observed that irradiation of a primary tumor in mice induced specific protection for 2–3 weeks against reinoculation of the tumor, while surgical removal of the tumor did not induce such immunologic protection. Moreover, it has been shown that cellular as well as humoral immune responses are radioresistant once they are initiated prior to irradiation [25, 34].

Finally, in some animal system, radiotherapy has a beneficial effect from the immunologic point of view. Some tumors act as depressors by diminishing the effectiveness of the cell-mediated response and by eliciting the production of blocking antibodies (antigen overexposure), and the larger the tumors the more pronounced the immunodepression. Nontreated tumor-bearing animals are immunologically inactive (immunologic eclipse). The immunologic reaction reappears after surgical removal. For that purpose, radiotherapy is as effective as surgery and also induces a significant reactivation [19]. O'TOOLE et al. [26] observed that lymphocyte cytotoxicity against urinary bladder cancer cells disappeared during the course of radiotherapy but reappeared within a matter of days. At Villejuif, LACOUR et al. carefully followed a few immunologic tests in patients with breast cancers receiving various types of treatment within the framework of a controlled clinical trial. They observed an improvement of immunologic reactions after local radiotherapy.

In conclusion, the so-called immunodepression caused by regional irradiation cannot be considered as a valid argument against the use of postoperative radiation therapy. Much more remains to be learned about the immune response relations to the various cancer treatments and to cancer survival before any worthy therapeutic generalization can be deduced from our knowledge.

Another supposed drawback of postoperative radiotherapy is the stimulation of subclinical metastases and surviving cells. In fact, an accelerated growth rate of the surviving cells of experimental tumors [22, 40] or human tumors [44, 23] has been observed after irradiation. The same phenomenon occurs after chemotherapy [31c] or surgical excision [31b] and is probably due to the reduction of tumor mass. It would be difficult to exclude any therapy of cancer for this reason. Furthermore, the practical importance of this phenomenon is very slight [43].

In summary, the supposed drawbacks of postoperative radiotherapy remain hypothetic, whereas the usefulness of prophylactic irradiation of clinically uninvolved areas has been proved for many types of cancer (head and neck, lymphoma, seminomas, medulloblastomas, etc.). During recent years, two new important developments have occurred:

1) Conservative treatment of small breast cancer (≤ 2–3 cm) in which tumorectomy is followed by local and regional irradiation. This is as effective as radical mastectomy and gives good cosmetic results. 2) Prophylactic irradiation of lungs for prevention of lung metastases has been shown effective. In the EORTC trial for osteosarcoma, it has significantly reduced the incidence of lung metastases without causing noticeable disturbance of lung function [5, and in this symposium].

References

1. Abbatucci, J. S.: L'irradiation pulmonaire de principe. Bases théoriques et expérience acquise. In: Pronostic et Traitement des Sarcomes Ostéogéniques. Trifaud, A., Meary, R. (eds.). Paris: Masson & Cie 1972

2. Abbatucci, J. S., Dutreix, A., Harichaux, P., Peyroux, J. P., Surmont, J., Tubiana, M.: Etude des modifications hématologiques consécutives à certaines techniques radiothérapiques. Ann. Radiol. (Paris) *1*, 365–379 (1958)
3. Alexander, P.: The bogey of the immunosuppressive action of local radiotherapy. Int. J. Radiat. Oncol. Biol. Phys. *1*, 369–371 (1976)
4. Blomgren, H., Berg, R., Wasserman, J., Glas, U.: Effect of radiotherapy on blood lymphocyte population in mammary carcinoma. Int. J. Radiat. Oncol. Biol. Phys. *1*, 177–188 (1976)
5. Breur, K., Cohen, P., Schweisguth, O., Hart, A. M. M.: Irradiation of the lungs as an adjuvant therapy of osteosarcoma of the limbs. An EORTC randomized study. Eur. J. Cancer *14*, 461–471 (1978)
6. Calle, R., Schlienger, P., Vilcoq, J. R.: Place et limite des thérapeutiques à visées conservatrices des épithéliomas mammaires. Résultats à 10 ans. Bull. Cancer (Paris) *64*, 633–648 (1977)
7. Cohen, L.: Theoretical iso-survival formulae for fractionated radiation therapy. Br. J. Radiol. *41*, 522–528 (1968)
8. Crile, G., Jr., Deodhar, S. D.: Role of pre-operative irradiation in prolonging concomitant immunity and preventing metastasis in mice. Cancer *27*, 629–634 (1971)
9. Easson, E. C.: Post-operative radiotherapy in breast cancer. In: Prognostic factors in breast cancer. Forrest, A. P. M., Kunkler, P. B. (eds.), pp. 118–127. Edinburgh: Livingstone 1968
10. Fisher, B., Slack, N. H., Cavanaugh, P. J., Gardner, B., Ravdin, R. G.: Post-operative radiotherapy in the treatment of breast cancer: results of the NSABP clinical trial. Ann. Surg. *172*, 711–732 (1970)
11. Fletcher, G. H.: Clinical dose-response curve of subclinical aggregates of epithelial cells. J. Radiol. Electrol. *53*, 201–206 (1972)
12. Fletcher, G. H.: Control by irradiation of peripheral lymphatic disease in breast cancer. Am. J. Roentgenol. *111*, 115–118 (1971)
13. Fletcher, G. H.: Elective irradiation of subclinical disease in cancers of the head and neck. Cancer *29*, 1450–1454 (1972)
14. Fu, K. K., Phillips, T. L., Wharam, M. D.: Radiation response of artificial pulmonary metastases of the EMT-6 tumor. Int. J. Radiat. Oncol. Biol. Phys. *1*, 257–260 (1976)
15. Frindel, E., Malaise, E. P., Alpen, E., Tubiana, M.: Kinetics of cell proliferation of an experimental tumor. Cancer Res. *27*, 1122–1131 (1967)
16. Glas, U., Wasserman, J.: Effect of radiation treatment on cellmediated immune response in carcinoma of the breast. Acta Radiol. [Ther.] (Stockh.) *13*, 83–94 (1974)
17. Hamilton, T., Langlands, A. O., Prescott, R. J.: The treatment of operable cancer of the breast: a clinical trial in the South-East region of Scotland. Br. J. Surg. *61*, 758–761 (1974)
18. Kaae, S., Johansen, H.: Simple versus radical mastectomy in primary breast cancer. In: Prognostic factors in breast cancer. Forrest, A. P. M., Kunkler, P. B. (eds.), pp. 93–102. Edinburgh: Livingstone 1968
19. Le Francois, D., Durán Troise, G., Chavaudra, N., Malaise, E., Barski, G.: Comparative effect of local radiotherapy and surgery on cellmediated immunity against a mouse transplantable tumor. Int. J. Cancer *13*, 629–639 (1974)
20. Levitt, S. H., McHugh, R. B., Song, C. W.: Radiotherapy in the post-operative treatment of operable cancer of the breast. II – A Re-examination of Stjernswärd's application of the Mantel-Haenszel statistical method. Evaluation of the effect of the radiation on the immune response and suggestions for post-operative radiotherapy. Cancer *39*, 933–940 (1976)
21. Little, J. B., Hahn, G. M., Frindel, E., Tubiana, M.: Repair of potentially lethal radiation damage in vitro and in vivo. Radiology *106*, 689–694 (1973)
22. Malaise, E., Tubiana, M.: Croissance des cellules d'un fibrosarcome expérimental irradié chez la souris C3H. C.R. Acad. Sci. [D] (Paris) *263*, 292–295 (1966)
23. Malaise, E., Charbit, A., Chavaudra, N., Combes, P. F., Douchez, J., Tubiana, M.: Chances in volume of irradiated human metastases. Investigation of repair of sublethal damage and tumour repopulation. Br. J. Cancer *26*, 43–52 (1972)

24a. McCredie, J. A., Inch, W. R., Sutherland, R. M.: Effect of postoperative radiotherapy on peripheral blood lymphocytes in patients with carcinoma of the breast. Cancer *29,* 349–356 (1972)

24b. Meyer, K. K.: Radiation induced lymphocyte immune deficiency. Arch. Surg. *101,* 114–121 (1970)

25. Nelson, A. J. III, Montague, E. D.: Resectable localized breast cancer. The rationale for combined surgery and irradiation. Jour. Am. Med. Assoc. *231,* 189–191 (1975)

26. O'Toole, C., Perlmann, P., Unsgaard, B., Almgård, L. E., Johansson, B., Moberger, G., Edsmyr, F.: Cellular immunity to human urinary bladder carcinoma. II – Effect of surgery and pre operative irradiation. Int. J. Cancer *10,* 92–98 (1972)

27. Sarrazin, D., Fontaine, F., Le, M., Mouriesse, H.: Données actuelles sur la radiothérapie du cancer du sein. Bull. Cancer (Paris) *62,* 373–390 (1975)

28. Schabel, F.: Concepts for systemic treatment of micrometastases. Cancer *35,* 15–24 (1975)

29. Shipley, W. U., Stanley, J. A., Steel, G. G.: Tumor size dependency in the radiation response of the Lewis lung carcinoma. Cancer Res. *35,* 2488–2493 (1975)

30. Shipley, W. U., Stanley, J. A., Courtenay, V. D., Field, S. B.: Repair of radiation damage in Lewis lung carcinoma cells following in situ treatment with fast neutrons and γ-rays. Cancer Res. *35,* 932–938 (1975)

31a. Shukovsky, L. J., Fletcher, G. H.: Time-dose and tumor volume relationships in the irradiation of squamous cell carcinoma of the tonsillar fossa. Radiology *107,* 621–626 (1973)

31b. Simpson-Herren, L., Sanford, A. H., Holmquist, J. P.: Effects of surgery on the cell kinetics of residual tumor. Cancer Treat. Rep. *60,* 1749–1760 (1976)

31c. Skipper, H. E.: Kinetic behaviour versus response to chemotherapy. Natl. Cancer Inst. Monogr. *34,* 2 (1971)

32. Steel, G. G., Adams, K.: Stem-cell survival and tumor control in the Lewis lung carcinoma. Cancer Res. *35,* 1530–1535 (1975)

33. Steel, G. G., Adams, K., Stanley, J.: Size dependence of the response of Lewis lung tumors to BCNU. Cancer Treat. Rep. *60,* 1743–1748 (1976)

34. Stewart, C. C., Perez, C. A.: Effect of irradiation on immune responses. Radiology *118,* 201–210 (1976)

35. Stjernswärd, J., Vanky, F., Jondal, M., Wigzell, H., Sealy, R.: Lymphopenia and change in distribution of human B and T lymphocytes in peripheral blood induced by irradiation for mammary carcinoma. Lancet *1,* 1352–1356 (1972)

36. Stjernswärd, J.: Decreased survival related to irradiation postoperatively in early operable breast cancer. Lancet *2,* 1285–1286 (1974)

37. Suit, H. D.: Introduction. In: Conference on time and dose relationships in radiation biology as applied to radiotherapy. Bond, V. P., Suit, H. D., Marcial, V. (eds.). Brookhaven National Laboratory Report BNL 50203 (C-57). Springfield, Va.: Clearinghouse for Federal Scientific and Technical Information 1970

38. Suit, H. D., Maeda, M.: Hyperbaric oxygen and radiobiology of a C3H mouse mammary carcinoma. J. Natl. Cancer Inst. *39,* 639–652 (1967)

39. Tapley, N. du V., Montague, E. D.: Elective irradiation with the electron beam after mastectomy for breast cancer. Am. J. Roentgenol. Rad. Ther. Nucl. Med. *126,* 127–134 (1976)

40. Tubiana, M., Frindel, E., Malaise, E. P.: The application of radiobiologic knowledge and cellular kinetics to radiation therapy. Am. J. Roentgenol. *102,* 822–830 (1968)

41. Tubiana, M., Lacour, J., Monnier, J. P., Bergiron, C., Gerard-Marchant, R., Roujeau, J., Bok, B., Parmentier, C.: External radiotherapy and radioactive iodine in the treatment of 359 thyroid cancers. Br. J. Radiol. *44,* 894–907 (1975)

42. Tubiana, M., Charbord, P., Cukersztein, W., Sarrazin, D., Fontaine, F., Parmentier, C.: The role of radiotherapy and radioactive iodine in the treatment of thyroid cancer without metastases. Ann. Radiol. *20,* 801–805 (1977)

43. Tubiana, M., Guichard, M., Malaise, E.: Determinants of cellular kinetics in radiotherapy. In: Growth kinetics and biochemical regulation of normal and malignant cells. Drewinko, B., Humphrey, R. M. (eds.), pp. 827–842. Baltimore: Williams & Wilkins 1977
44. Van Peperzeel, H. A.: Effects of single doses of radiation on lung metastases in man and experimental animals. Eur. J. Cancer *8,* 665–675 (1972)
45. Wallgren, A., De Schryver, A., Wasserman, J.: L'essai de Stockholm de radiothérapie préopératoire dans le cancer du sein opérable. Bull. Cancer *64,* 627–631 (1977)

Possible Drawback of Radiotherapy: Rational and Experimental Bases of Post-Surgical Therapies

J. Stjernswärd

Radiotherapy has a clear role in the management of secondary spread. It is used for elective treatment of subclinical disease in defined high-risk groups, for palliation of clinical metastases, to reach secondary spread in anatomically, pharmacologically, or immunologically privileged sanctuaries, as a cytotoxic agent in total body irradiation, and lately in combination therapy with chemotherapy. Radiotherapy has a demonstrated positive role in the control of secondary spread, despite being a localized form of therapy and although distant metastases represent the major cause of failure in cancer therapy, except for tumors of the central nervous system and head and neck. A new era of multidisciplinary approach, based on knowledge of the biology of the tumor, is here and the role of radiotherapy in a combined modality approach needs reevaluation in an attempt to explore the optimal effectiveness of each treatment method: surgery, radiotherapy, chemotherapy, hormone therapy, and perhaps also immunotherapy. Much remains to be understood about how these different treatment modalities work in synergism of antagonism with each other and their optimal timing and combination so as not to over- or undertreat the patient. The old hierarchic approach of first the surgeon, then the radiotherapist, then the endocrinologist, and finally the chemotherapist should be replaced by an initial management decision including all the various disciplines working cooperatively.

Radiotherapy, like other treatment modalities, is not exempt from the assumption that it may have negative side-effects. This analysis of possible drawbacks of radiotherapy will thus be limited to possible negative side-effects, especially those that might occur when radiotherapy is combined with systemic therapies for minimal residual disease in a modern multimodality approach. Possible drawbacks of adjuvant radiotherapy, are:

1. Overtreatment: priority should be given to systemic therapies of certain diseases, and routine postoperative irradiation is overtreatment;
2. Compromise of systemic therapies;
3. Delay of systemic therapies;
4. Geographic miss (when the biology of the tumor is ignored).

It cannot at the moment be excluded that adjuvant radiotherapy may *compromise* the effect of systemic therapies under certain circumstances. More is not necessarily always better where therapies are concerned. This is indicated by data on testis cancer, where the response to chemotherapy, which unlike radiotherapy can have a curative effect in disseminated disease, was compromised if the patient had been irradiated [5]. Holland [1] has given data comparing results in operable breast cancer patients with four or more axillary lymph nodes positive for tumor and receiving a Cooper adjuvant chemotherapy regimen with irradiation and those receiving chemotherapy alone, showing that those irradiated had more disease relapses than the chemotherapy only group: 13 of 27 patients who received chemotherapy and irradiation relapsed, compared with 6 of 73 with chemotherapy only. One of the many possible explanations for this finding may be a negative systemic effect of irradiation, counterbalancing the systemic effect of chemotherapy. The two groups were biologically balanced, except that the mean numbers of positive axillary lymph nodes were 7.7 in the chemotherapy only group as against 9.3 in the chemotherapy + irradiation group. If a difference of 1.6 positive lymph nodes is biologically important this may be another explanation for the high failure risk seen when irradiation was added. The data of the Scandinavian adjuvant chemotherapy group [4] indicate that when monochemotherapy was *delayed* due to irradiation, the positive effect observed when monochemotherapy is given around the time of operation to operable breast cancer patients did not occur.

Systemic side-effects of irradiation that definitively influence the outcome of subsequent chemotherapy are demonstrated elegantly in a careful analysis by the MRC Working Party on Leukemia in Childhood [2, 3, 13]. The working party showed that modifications of chemotherapy after cranial irradiation were significant and the significance was related to whether or not the patient died in complete remission during the first weeks after CNS irradiation due to infectious disease [2]. The lymphopenia induced by treatment for acute lymphoblastic leukemia (ALL) has been analyzed and discussed in relation to the type and incidence of infection occurring in patients dying during complete remission [3, 13]. In patients with ALL, radiotherapy will be given priority, as it reaches cells in privileged sanctuaries, and the chemotherapy has to be modified accordingly. However, for solid tumors, e.g., testis cancer, as indicated by data already mentioned [5], priority for radiotherapy will not be the case. Due to negative side-effects of irradiation in these cases, chemotherapy should have priority over irradiation, which perhaps should even be avoided as a routine form of treatment.

A severe drawback of radiotherapy used in the classic way, i.e., as a routine postoperative treatment modality, is that a high number of patients are unnecessarily treated, in fact they are *overtreated.* This is exemplified in operable node-positive breast cancer patients: *routine* postoperative irradiation to node-positive patients does not prolong survival [6, 9]. More is not necessarily better. Simple logic would seem enough to stop the use of irradiation routinely in operable cancer [8]. Furthermore, results from multiple drug chemotherapy trials show that soft tissue recurrences, which are the primary target for the irradiation, are precisely the tumors that will respond best to systemic multiple drug chemotherapy [10]. Irradiation, as opposed to chemotherapy, has only a locoregional tumor-neutralizing effect. Thus although both may have systemic side-effects, chemotherapy may also affect the systemic disease.

The question of whether the *facilitation of metastases* found in experimental animal tumors is relevant to the human situation is still open [7, 12]. Results showing that nidation and/or local outgrowth of tumor cells may be facilitated in irradiated human tissues are documented [11]. Over the last 20 years, more than 4000 patients with operable breast cancer and hundreds of patients with stage I ovarian cancer have been investigated in clinical controlled trials (breast) and documented (ovarian) in research reports, in which the main difference was whether or not the patients received postoperative radiotherapy [10, 11]. There is concordance between these clinical data and the experimental data that show increased dissemination of disease after irradiation. Experience with human breast and ovarian cancer indicates that prophylactic irradiation of the tumor bed after complete removal of the primary tumor does not increase survival, and on the contrary, when there is a high frequency of occult disseminated disease outside the irradiated target volume, it may even be harmful [9, 11, 12]. Few doubt the positive effect of irradiation when the tumor is in the right target volume, but this is an example of "geographic miss," as the significant tumor masses deciding the outcome are outside the irradiated volume, as shown by Mangioni and Morasca by peritoneoscopy at this meeting. In both examples mentioned above, there are frequently distant micrometastases outside the

Table 1. Survival in ovarian cancer (stage I) with and without postoperative irradiation[a]

Study	Survival at 5 years (%)		Mortality in irradiated groups compared with surgery only (%)	No. of patients at start of study	
	Surgery only	Surgery + radiotherapy		Surgery only	Surgery + radiotherapy
Decreased survival					
Rubin et al.	91	62	+ 29	11	12
Maus et al.	66.7	57.9	+ 8.8	33	28
Munnell	78	53	+ 24	98	81
Munnell	80	54	+ 26	20	35
Dalley	88	67	+ 21	8	12
Barr et al.	72	65	+ 7	40	17
Bagley et al.	63	66	− 3		
Bagley et al.	70	50	+ 20		
Webb et al.	89.3	73.4	+ 15.9	105	98
Webb et al.	88.2	52	+ 36.2	43	25
Clark et al.	60	53	+ 7	46	101
Increased survival					
Kent et al.	46.4	71.1	− 24	69	45

[a] Adapted from [11]. Please see [11] for detailed references regarding studies quoted.

irradiated target volume, as confirmed by later mortality. The use of routine irradiation postoperatively in such a situation offers the possibility of analyzing whether the biologic mechanism documented in animal models showing an increased frequency of metastases after irradiation also exists in humans. Table 1 shown that adding postoperative irradiation to the treatment of stage I ovarian cancer certainly does not prolong survival. The 5-year mortality is higher in the irradiated group in most studies. It is difficult to analyze these data, but they hardly support the continued use of irradiation postoperatively in stage I ovarian cancer.

All the breast cancer studies referred to are prospective, randomized, and controlled. The ovarian studies are retrospective. A high degree of patient selection cannot be excluded in the latter. It cannot be ruled out completely that clinical intuition about prognosis within the same stage of disease in ovarian cancer has given a larger survival difference than that between classified stages of disease after pathologic staging. It is an open question whether the radiotherapists' explanation for the observed increased mortality in the irradiated group is due to this or due to the fact that postoperative radiotherapy as a treatment modality may be a factor that can explain the difference. It cannot be excluded that the increased mortality usually observed after the addition of postoperative radiotherapy in ovarian stage I cancer may be due to the treatment modality itself [11]. The more conventional explanation is that this may be due to patient selection within the same stage of disease, but the data may reflect an interesting biologic mechanism of importance in explaining the increased frequency of metastases after irradiation, in parallel with mechanisms found in experimental animal systems. Some possible mechanisms explaining the increased frequency of metastases after irradiation have been summarized elsewhere [12].

In conclusion, radiotherapy is not exempt from the requirement that our different treatment modalities should be assessed by means of the data available from properly designed trials. Like most treatment modalities, radiotherapy has certain drawbacks. Used wisely, however, the therapeutic advantages of radiotherapy dominate.

References

1. Holland, J. F.: Therapy of primary breast cancer. Isr. J. Med. Sci. 829–836 (1977)
2. MacLennan, I. C. M., Peto, J., Kay, H. E. M.: Analysis of treatment in childhood leukaemia. V. Advantage of reduced chemotherapy during and immediately after cranial irradiation. Br. J. Cancer *36,* 625–633 (1977)
3. MacLennan, I. C. M., Kay, H. E. M., Festenstein, M., Smith, P. G.: Analysis of treatment in childhood leukaemia. I. Predisposition to methotrexate-induced neutropenia after craniospinal irradiation. Report to the Medical Research Council of the Working Party on Leukaemia in Childhood. Br. Med. J. *3,* 563–566 (1975)
4. Nissen-Meyer, R., Kjellgren, K., Malmio, K., Mansson, B., Norin, N.: Surgical adjuvant chemotherapy. Results with one short course with cyclophosphamide after mastectomy for breast cancer. Cancer (in press) (1978)
5. Samuels, M. L., Lanzotti, V. J., Holoye, P. Y., Boyle, L. E., Smith, T. L., Johnson, D. E.: Combination chemotherapy in germinal cell tumors. Cancer Treat. Rev. *3,* 185–204 (1976)
6. Stjernswärd, J.: Decreased survival correlated to local irradiation in "early" operable breast cancer. Lancet *1974 II,* 1285–1286
7. Stjernswärd, J.: Radiotherapy and metastatic spread. In: New aspects of breast cancer. Vol. 3: Secondary spread in breast cancer. Stoll, B. A. (ed.), Chapter 9, pp. 139–167. London: Heinemann Medical and Yearbook Publishers 1977
8. Stjernswärd, J.: Radiotherapy in the therapeutic strategy to breast cancer. Recent Results Cancer Res. *62,* 127–133 (1977)
9. Stjernswärd, J.: Can survival be decreased by post-operative irradiation. Int. J. Radiat. Oncol. Biol. Phys. *2,* 1171–1175 (1977)
10. Stjernswärd, J.: Adjuvant radiotherapy trials in breast cancer. A report to the profession, Washington 1976. Cancer *39,* 2846–2867 (1977)
11. Stjernswärd, J., Douglas, P.: Immunosuppression and metastasis. In: Cancer invasion and metastasis: biologic mechanisms and therapy. Day, S. B. et al. (eds.), pp. 311–323. New York: Raven Press 1977
12. von Essen, C. F., Stjernswärd, J.: Radiotherapy and metastases. In: Secondary spread of cancer. Baldwin, R., (ed.), Chapter III, pp. 73–99. New York, London: Academic Press 1978
13. Waller, C. A., MacLennan, I. C. M., Campbell, A. C., Festenstein, M., Kay, H. E. M.: Medical Research Council's Working Party on Leukaemia in Childhood: Analysis of treatment in childhood leukaemia. III. Independence of lymphopenia induced by irradiation and by chemotherapy. Br. J. Haematol. *35,* 597–612 (1977)

Adjuvant Chemotherapy: Theoretical Considerations and Model Studies[1]

L. M. van Putten, J. de Ruiter, C. J. H. van de Velde, J. H. Mulder, and A. F. C. Gerritsen

Introduction

In his presentation at the previous meeting on adjuvant therapy in Tucson, FREI [6] concluded that the effectiveness of adjuvant chemotherapy could very simply be derived from a consideration of four parameters: sensitivity of the tumor to each treatment course, the growth rate of the tumor, the number of treatment courses, and the interval between the courses. He used a formula of the following type:

$$\text{Total log tumor cell kill} = (\log K) \times N - \frac{\log 2}{DT} \times (N-1) \times I$$

in which K is the cell kill per course, N the number of courses, I the interval between them, and DT the tumor doubling time during regrowth between treatments. Although this formula is undoubtedly valid, its usefulness is limited to a comparison of different treatment intensities to similar tumors. In this sense it was applied to the treatment of osteosarcoma and gave useful insight into the effect of different treatments. In contrast, comparison of the sensitivity of different types of tumors or prediction of response is not feasible since we do not know the parameters K and DT. They are likely to vary from tumor to tumor and since no data are available to help us here, we have considered as a first approximation that these parameters might be similar or proportional for primary tumors and for residual disease. This would imply that the success of adjuvant chemotherapy might be predictable from the results obtained with a similar treatment applied to manifest disease.

It is the purpose of this paper to present data on experimental studies in which effects on primary tumors can be compared with the effect on residual disease. It is, however, impossible to use cell kill as a parameter for comparison since the data are not available and for this reason tumor growth delay or survival was used.

Most data are available on Lewis lung tumor; its tendency to early metastasis after subcutaneous or intramuscular inoculation has been widely used and many data are available to indicate that the metastatic disease is much more sensitive than the primary tumor to single-drug [8, 9] or combination [10] chemotherapy. This increased sensitivity is explained by:

a) The smaller cell number that makes elimination of the tumor easier (especially if the number of metastases is used as the endpoint);
b) The larger fraction of cells in cycle and the higher rate of proliferation, which increases drug sensitivity;
c) The absence of necrotic areas in small metastases, which diminishes the release of metabolites competing with some cytostatic drugs;
d) The higher drug levels observed in small metastatic foci compared to larger primary tumors [5].

---

1 Supported by the Koningin Wilhelmina Fonds, Netherlands Organization for the Fight against Cancer.

It is, therefore, not surprising that increased sensitivity of minimal disease has been found in other tumors. SCHABEL [12] has presented data on C3H mammary tumors, B16 melanoma, and colon tumor 26 indicating a much longer prolongation of survival if therapy is applied to residual disease than if applied to larger primary tumors.

Our own experiences are, however, quite different. A number of studies were devoted to the metastasizing mammary carcinoma 2661 described by VAN DE VELDE [14]. He noted a growth delay of flank tumors after CMF combination of 36 days, but when the same treatment was given to mice with residual disease after surgery the delay of death was only 18 days. This suggests that the residual disease is less sensitive than the large primary tumor, but growth delay is not an absolute parameter for effectiveness; an equal log cell kill may be associated with less growth delay for rapidly growing minimal tumors than for a large tumor (Fig. 1). Further experiments with this tumor have, however, confirmed our suspicions that the metastatic disease is less responsive than the primary tumor. In the first place, it was demonstrated that certain dose levels of CMF treatment actually caused earlier death from metastatic spread than observed in animals treated with surgery alone (Table 1 and Fig. 2). In the second place, treatment of flank tumors with the same drug combination actually permitted cure of a significant number of mice (Fig. 3). From these results, it must be concluded that the discrepancy is real and that indeed the treatment of minimal disease is less effective than the treatment of a large flank tumor. As evident from Table 1; the response is more favorable if the survival time after surgery alone is short, indicating that paradoxically larger quantities of residual disease seem to respond relatively better.

It is notable that in the adjuvant therapy studies lymph node localization of the disease was always clearly sensitive to the chemotherapy, whereas the pulmonary localization seemed to

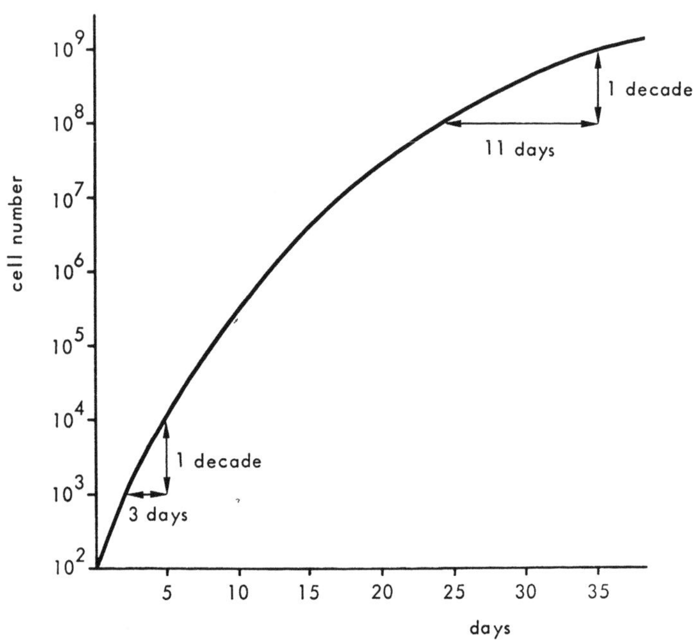

Fig. 1. A tumor that is growing progressively slower will respond with different times of growth delay, depending on its size, when treated with a dose of chemotherapy that causes 1 decade of cell killing

Table 1. Median survival time after tumor cell inoculation in the foot pad, amputation of the primary tumor on day 10, and various intensities of CMF[a] chemotherapy for 4 weeks

	Days (No. of mice)			
	Surgery alone	Surgery + 1 CMF	Surgery + ¾ CMF	Surgery + ½ CMF
Exp. 1	25 (7)	43 (13)[b]		
Exp. 2	77 (19)	101 (5)	56 (10)[c]	59 (10)[c]
Exp. 3	> 74 (19)	> 66 (10)	52 (19)	> 74 (10)
Exp. 4	45 (14)	71 (12)		
Mice dying from drug toxicity have been eliminated				

[a] For dosages of this treatment see legend of Fig. 2.
[b] Significantly different from surgery alone; $P < 0.05$.
[c] Significantly different from surgery alone; $P < 0.025$.

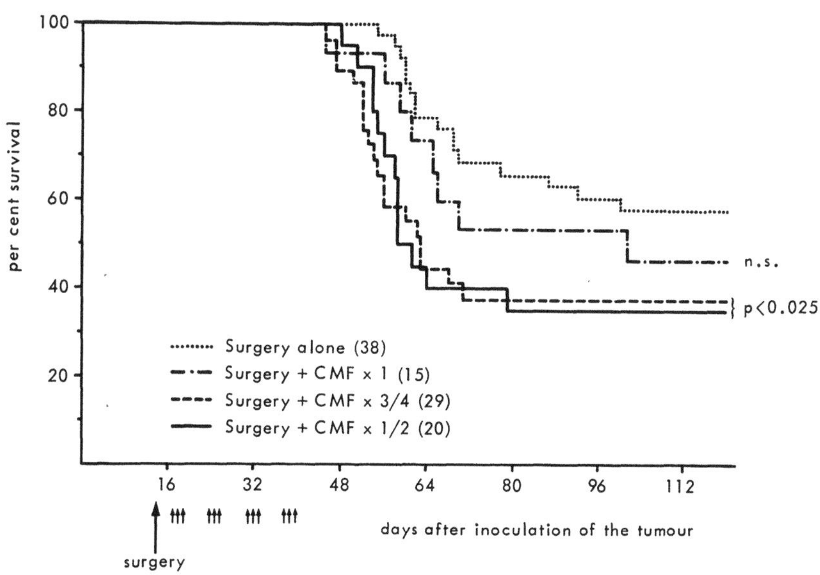

Fig. 2. Carcinoma 2661 was inoculated into the foot pad of mice on day 0. The tumor-bearing leg was amputated on day 14. Three days later, different groups of mice were given either no adjuvant chemotherapy or combination chemotherapy (CMF) consisting of four weekly schedules of: cyclophosphamide 3 days 100 mg/m^2, methotrexate 30 mg/m^2 on day 1, and 5-fluorouracil 300 mg/m^2 on day 1. (This schedule was extrapolated directly from the dosage used in man per 4-week course). One group each received this treatment in full dosage, at three-quarters or at one-half the listed dosages. The number of mice in each group are given in brackets. It is evident that the treatment decreases survival although drug-induced death from toxicity (before day 45) has been eliminated

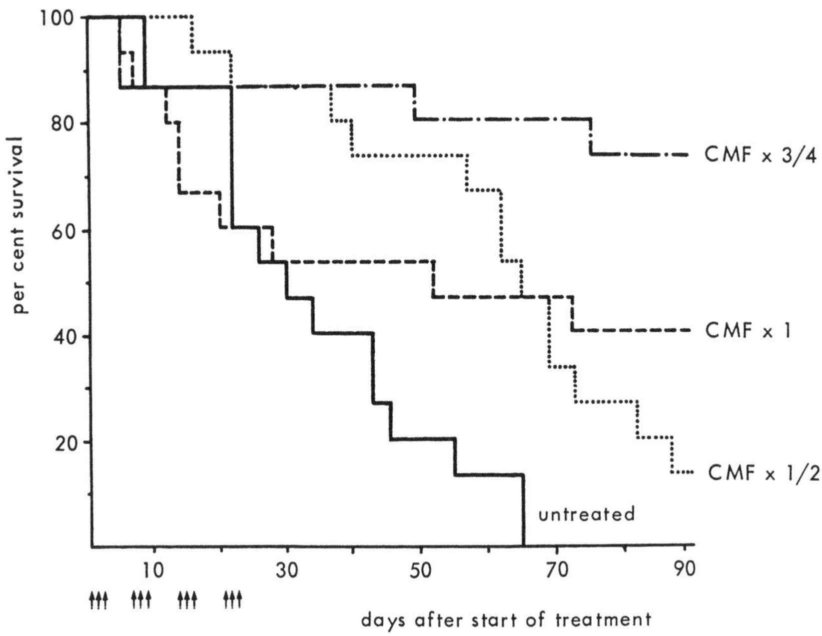

Fig. 3. Treatment of mice carrying flank tumors with a similar schedule as was used for postoperative adjuvant therapy in Fig. 2. The flank tumor responds markedly to the treatment, and cures were observed (in this case, drug-induced death from toxicity is responsible for part of the early mortality in the group: CMF × 1)

be hardly affected by the drug treatment. This was initially observed to occur in mice dying spontaneously from recurrent disease [14]. Since it was conceivable that the variation in survival time could have influenced these results, a similar study was carried out on mice sacrificed specifically for evaluation of the distribution of recurrent disease after adjuvant therapy. The results are presented in Table 2. It is obvious that there is no significant difference in pulmonary tumors with and without adjuvant therapy, whereas the lymph nodes

Table 2. Effect of adjuvant chemotherapy with cyclophosphamide, methotrexate and 5-fluorouracil on the distribution of recurrent disease

Treatment	Number of lung metastases per mouse		Mice with lymph node metastasis	
	Mean ± SD	Median	Incidence	%
Controls	27.5 ± 60.9	1	12/18	67
Four weeks CMF chemotherapy	7.6 ± 9.2	4	1/11	9
Significance	N.S.		$P < 0.01$	

Mice were inoculated with tumor 2661 in the foot pad (day 0); the foot was amputated on day 18/19. Four weeks of chemotherapy started on day 21. The mice were sacrificed on day 57.

are markedly less affected in the drug-treated mice. A similar difference in response between different localizations of tumor growth has been described for spontaneous mammary tumors in mice [7] in which postsurgical chemotherapy was effective in suppressing local recurrences without significantly affecting metastatic spread. Differences in response to chemotherapy of different localizations of metastatic disease are well-known to clinicians; for instance, visceral and skin lesions in malignant melanoma differ markedly in sensitivity to cytostatic therapy. Also the discrepancy between treatment effectiveness on minimal disease and large tumors observed in our model is seen in patients; the difference in effect of adjuvant therapy on pre- and postmenopausal breast cancer is not paralleled by a similar difference in effectiveness of treatment of recurrent breast cancer (Compare the data of BONADONNA et al. [1] and DE LENA et al. [3] with a similar treatment schedule in both conditions). From this we may conclude that neither models nor clinical studies support the concept that the success of adjuvant chemotherapy may consistently be predicted from the effect of treatment of recurrent disease.

Mechanisms

To explain the lower efficacy of adjuvant therapy on minimal disease in our model, a number of hypotheses have been considered. In the first place, immunosuppression by the chemotherapy could be ruled out. The tumor used in these studies is nonimmunogenic as confirmed in repeated studies by different methods [14]. A second possibility has received more attention. It involves the aspecific host resistance that was found to occur against growth of (pseudometastatic) tumor nodules in the lung after intravenous inoculation. This resistance may be abolished by cyclophosphamide as described both for poorly immunogenic tumors [2, 4, 13, 15] and for markedly antigenic tumors [11]. In the latter, the effect seems to be quantitatively less important. The effect of cyclophosphamide is especially obvious if the drug is given shortly (1–4 days) before inoculation of the tumor cells, but recently a similar effect on host resistance was also shown to operate when the drug was given after tumor cell inoculation [16]. This possibility was seriously considered by us, but two sets of data argue against it. Attempts were made to obtain a cyclophosphamide-resistant cell line from tumor 2661 since this might show more clearly the presence of a growth-promoting effect of cyclophosphamide on the spontaneously metastasizing tumor in the absence of a simultaneous cell-killing effect. As shown in Table 3, this tumor line 2661/Cy did indeed show a very limited response to doses

Table 3. Effects of treatment with cyclophosphamide on the insensitive subline of tumor 2661

	Growth delay of primary tumor (days)	Median survival time (days) after chemotherapy, given	
		Before surgery	After surgery
Control	–	65 44 65	62
1 × 200 mg/kg cyclophosphamide	2.0; – 0.5; 1.8	62[a] 79[a]	71[a]
4 × 50 mg/kg cyclophosphamide	2.3[b]	> 120 > 140[a]	75[a]

[a] Significant difference in death rate as calculated by logrank test.
[b] $p = 0.025$.

of cyclophosphamide, which markedly delayed growth of the original tumor line. When given either before of after surgery for the primary tumor, cyclophosphamide failed completely to show a tumor growth-promoting effect; it showed even a significant therapeutic effect. Thus, our "resistant" tumor cell line showed the type of response known to occur in Lewis lung tumor and many others, which respond much better when exposed as minimal disease than as a large flank tumor, and the treatment resistance of the original line could not be identified in this subline.

Another argument against aspecific host resistance as a mechanism explaining the poor response of our mammary carcinoma to adjuvant treatment may be found in the fact that marked host resistance has been found to occur in Lewis lung tumor [17], which nevertheless appears to show high sensitivity to adjuvant chemotherapy. In conclusion, our attempts to explain the resistance of minimal disease to adjuvant chemotherapy in our model tumor 2661 as either due to immunosuppression or to the suppression of aspecific host resistance have not met with success and alternative explanations must be studied. Experimental analysis of this mechanism is of importance since this tumor shares with clinically observed tumors the property of a response to adjuvant chemotherapy that is much less than expected on the basis of effects observed on large primary tumors.

Summary

Comparison of response of experimental tumors to adjuvant chemotherapy for minimal disease with the response of solid large tumors to similar drug regimens has indicated that for many tumors the small microscopic foci are more responsive. There are, however, a number of model tumors that respond far less to chemotherapy when applied to minimal disease than when applied to large tumors. The response of these tumors to adjuvant treatment shows similarities with the clinically observed response. The data do not support the hypothesis that the success of a drug combination given as adjuvant chemotherapy may be predicted from the success of the same treatment when applied for manifest disease.

References

1. Bonadonna, G., Rossi, A., Valagussa, P., Banfi, A., Veronesi, U.: The CMF program for operable breast cancer with positive axillary nodes. Cancer *39*, 2904–2915 (1977)
2. Carmel, R. J., Brown, J. M.: The effect of cyclophosphamide and other drugs on the incidence of pulmonary metastases in mice. Cancer *37*, 145–151 (1977)
3. De Lena, M., Brambilla, C., Morabito, A., Bonadonna, G.: Adriamycin plus vincristine compared to and combined with cyclophosphamide, methotrexate and 5-fluorouracil for advanced breast cancer. Cancer *35*, 1108–1115 (1975)
4. De Ruiter, J., Smink, T., Van Putten, L. M.: Studies on the enhancement by cyclophosphamide of artificial lung metastasis after labeled cell inoculation. Cancer Treat. Rep. *60*, 465–470 (1976)
5. Donelli, M. G., Garattini, S.: Differential accumulation of anticancer agents in metastases compared with primary tumors in experimental models. In: Recent advances in cancer treatment. Tagnon, H. J., Staquet, M. (eds.), p. 177. New York: Raven Press 1977
6. Frei, E., Jaffe, N., Skipper, H. E., Gero, M. G.: Adjuvant chemotherapy of osteogenic sarcoma: progress and prospectives. In: Adjuvant therapy of cancer. Salmon, S. S., Jones, S. E. (eds.), p. 49. Amsterdam, New York: North Holland 1977

7. Fugman, R. A., Anderson, J. C., Stolfi, R. L., Martin, D. S.: Comparison of adjuvant chemotherapy against primary and metastatic spontaneous murine tumours. Cancer Res. *30*, 496–500 (1977)
8. Hellman, K., Salsbury, A. J., Burrage, K. S., Le Serve, A. W., James, S. E.: Drug induced inhibition of hematogeneously spread metastasis. In: Chemotherapy of cancer spread and metastasis. Garattini, S., Franchi, G. (eds.), p. 355. New York: Raven Press 1973
9. Karrer, K., Humphreys, S. R.: Continuous and limited courses of cyclophosphamide in mice with pulmonary metastasis after surgery. Cancer Chemother. Rep. *51*, 439–449 (1967)
10. Mulder, J. H., Smink, T., Van Putten, L. M.: Schedule dependent effectiveness of CCNU and 5-fluorouracil in experimental chemotherapy. Eur. J. Cancer *13*, 1123–1131 (1977)
11. Peters, L. J., Mason, K.: Enhancement of artificial lung metastases by cyclophosphamide: Pharmacological and mechanistic considerations. In: Cancer invasion and metastasis: Biologic mechanisms and therapy. Day, S. B., et al. (eds.). New York: Raven Press 1977
12. Schabel, F. M.: Surgical adjuvant chemotherapy of metastatic murine tumors. Cancer *40*, 558–568 (1977)
13. Steel, G. G., Adams, K.: Enhancement by cytostatic agents of artificial pulmonary metastasis. Br. J. Cancer *36*, 653–658 (1977)
14. van de Velde, C. J. H., van Putten, L. M., Zwaveling, A.: A new metastasizing mammary carcinoma model in mice: model characteristics and applications. Eur. J. Cancer *13*, 555–565 (1977)
15. van Putten, L. M., Kram, L. K. J., van Dierendonck, H. H. C., Smink, T., Füzy, M.: Enhancement by drugs of metastatic lung nodule formation after intravenous tumour cell injection. Int. J. Cancer *15*, 588–595 (1975)
16. van Putten, L. M.: Cell cycle specificity of anticancer agents. In: Fundamentals of Cancer Chemotherapy. Antibiotics Chemother. *23*, 128–134 (1978)
17. van Putten, L. M.: (to be published)

Design of Adjuvant Chemotherapy Based on Target Cell Determinants of Drug Action: Possibilities and Limitations[1]

Y. Rustum, Y. C. Cheng, Z. Pavelic, P. Creaven, and E. Mihich

Introduction

The traditional approach to surgical adjuvant chemotherapy is to select a drug or combination of drugs that have been shown to be effective against advanced disease of the tumor type being treated and to use them in a prospective randomized clinical trial. Such trials frequently involve a large number of patients treated over several years. Another conceptual approach is discussed herein, namely attempting to predict at the time of surgery the specific sensitivity of the tumor and to treat each patient with chemotherapy designed for that individual. Such an approach is in its infancy and may finally prove logistically impracticable, but its conceptual appeal is such that at this time it must be pursued so that its validity may be verified.

At the present state of knowledge it seems reasonable to assume that the selective toxicity of anticancer drugs depends on a multiplicity of factors [3]. Indeed, the action of a drug in target cells may be determined by such factors as (1) binding to, and transport through, the plasma membrane, (2) activation inside the cell or a cell compartment, (3) regulatory mechanisms at the proximal site of action potentially leading to adaptation of repair, (4) the cascade of changes that take place as a result of the perturbation of a network of enzymes within a close metabolic pathway and the influence on these changes exerted by intracellular or extracellular factors through modifications in metabolite pools, (5) the rate of decrease of active drug concentration in the cell, (6) the metabolic requirements of the target cell as related to cell function or kinetics, and (7) the effects of agents administered concurrently. In addition to determinants that operate primarily in the target cell population, drug kinetics and metabolic disposition in the whole body may affect cellular toxicity inasmuch as they determine drug or active metabolite availability to target cells as a function of time. Homeostatic mechanisms such as hormonal influences may also modify the metabolism of target cells and thus affect their sensitivity to a drug. It is, therefore, not surprising that a great deal of individual variability in response to a drug is commonly observed among patients with the same histopathologic and clinical type of tumor.

Adjuvant chemotherapy is defined for the purpose of this discussion as the postsurgical treatment of clinically undetectable residual disease. Despite the obvious major differences in pathophysiology between solid tumors and leukemias, in terms of design of chemotherapeutic strategies, certain similarities may be assumed to exist. Thus, for example, the so-called remission consolidation and maintenance treatments of acute leukemias may have characteristics and prerequisites that may not be too different from those of adjuvant postsurgical treatments. Any possible analogy, however, should take into consideration the fact that, in the case of solid tumors, residual disease is likely to be in the form of micrometastasis that would have the vascularization and stroma characteristics of a solid tumor, in contrast to the

---

1 The data from this Center discussed were obtained in studies supported in part by USPHS Grants CA-13038, CA-18420, CA-21071, CA-5834 and CA-18499.

predominant single-cell type physiology of leukemic reservoirs or disseminated cell populations.

Keeping in mind the basic concept that selectivity of drug action is likely to be determined by a multiplicity of integrated biochemical and pharmacologic factors for each drug and tumor, it may be possible to identify a relatively limited set of parameters, which may represent the summation of diversified events and which may allow a prediction of the sensitivity of individual patients to that drug. At this time the value of measurements of target cell determinants of drug action for a prediction of sensitivity of human tumors is in most cases relatively uncertain. Nevertheless, the initial experience gained with arabinosylcytosine (araC), adriamycin, and a few other agents in patients with leukemia is promising enough to encourage further studies not only in these diseases but also in patients with solid tumors. Because of the possible gross analogies mentioned above, the information obtained in patients with acute myelocytic leukemia (AML) may represent a starting point toward the development of concepts applicable to the design of strategies useful in adjuvant chemotherapy.

Experience Gained with araC in Patients with AML

In initial studies [6], the uptake of araC and the formation and retention of araCTP in target cells were compared to therapeutic efficacy in three murine tumor systems. The occurrence of similar plasma kinetics of intact drug ($t_{1/2}$ of about 20 min) in the three model systems studied excluded a differential role of these factors in the effects observed. Therapeutic efficacy against leukemias L1210 and P288 and Taper hepatoma was measured as percent increase in life span and incidence of 60-day survivors. Treatment was given intraperitoneally 1 day after the intraperitoneal inoculation of 10^6 tumor cells; the effects of a single drug administration (120 mg/kg) were compared to those of repeated administrations over a 24-h period. The formation and retention of araCTP were studied by measuring intracellular araCTP concentrations, 15, 60, 120, and 240 min after the intravenous injection of 20 μCi of araC-5-^{3}H (25 mg/kg) to ip tumor-bearing mice. Parallel araCTP retention measurements were performed after 30 min in vitro incubation of tumor cells with 10 μCi of [^{3}H]araC(1×10^{-6} *M*). The intracellular amount of araCTP formed in vivo or in vitro was greatest in L1210 cells, lowest in Taper hepatoma cells, and intermediate in P288 cells. In L1210 cells the highest level was reached at 15 min and was then only slightly reduced over a 4-h period. In Taper hepatoma and P288 cells, the highest levels of araCTP were reached at 60 min and then rapidly decreased, with only traces being left in Taper hepatoma cells at 4 h. The amount of araUMP formed in the three tumors was small and comparable; the araCMP pools were larger in Taper hepatoma than in the other two cell lines. The therapeutic efficacy of araC (e.g., at the dose of 20 mg/kg Q4 h × 6) was greatest against L1210 (ILS 158% with 8/15 mice were 60-day survivors), nil against Taper hepatoma, and moderate against P288 (ILS 68% with no long-term survivors), thus showing a good correlation with araCTP retention in the corresponding target cells [6]. The intracellular concentration of dCTP, the metabolite competing with araCTP, was comparable in the three tumors [8] and thus was not correlated with therapeutic response. In view of the correlation between intracellular araCTP retention and sensitivity to araC in murine model systems [6], it was argued that this parameter may provide a useful predictive index of target cell sensitivity, and perhaps clinical response, in human leukemia.

In a series of 28 previously untreated patients with AML, the formation and 4-h retention of araCTP in purified bone marrow leukemic myeloblasts incubated in vitro for 30 min with labeled araC (7.0×10^{-7} *M*) were measured in accordance with the design of the experiments previously performed in mice [9]. In terms of 4-h araCTP retention, the 28 patients fell into two major groups, namely those whose cells had a mean retention of 7.5 ± 4.2 pmol/10^7 cells and those whose cells had a retention of 0.32 ± 0.30 pmol/10^7 cells. A close correlation was found between retention and duration of complete remission (CR): 50% of patients with high retention were in CR at 140 weeks and 50% of patients with low retention were in CR at 30 weeks. Comparable studies were also carried out by others [1]. The good correlation evidenced in these studies is in contrast to the lack of correlation between clinical response and ratio of araC phosphorylation to deamination rates [10].
In addition to the findings with araC, results obtained with 3-deazauridine [2, 7] suggest the possibility that, at least in human leukemia and for certain drugs, appropriate indices and determinants of drug action, in most cases representing a summation of integrated phenomena, may indeed be identified and may provide a basis for a reliable prediction of response. The question should be asked, therefore, whether similar approaches could be fruitfully pursued in the case of certain solid tumors.

Initial Leads in Patients with Solid Tumors

Even before attempting to verify the validity of this approach to the design of specific chemotherapy of patients with solid tumors, one should ask four sets of fundamental questions. These may be formulated as follows:

1. Is there sufficient variability among individual patients in terms of critical target tumor metabolic features as to be responsible for a major variability in response to a drug or set of drugs;
2. Does this variability justify measuring presumed metabolic determinants of drug action in efforts to predict the potentiality for response;
3. Would it be possible on the basis of such measurements not only to predict the potentiality for response but also to design optimal chemotherapy for the individual patient;
4. Is it reasonable to assume that the technical difficulties in design and sampling intrinsic to studies in patients with solid tumors may be overcome so that the overall approach is truly feasible.

Most of these questions cannot yet be answered, and indeed most of them are still open even in the case of leukemias; nevertheless, at the present state of knowledge, major efforts are clearly warranted toward obtained information that may provide some of the needed answers and hopefully may also represent initial steps toward pursuing further the field of clinical research under consideration. The results of some of the preliminary studies carried out in this laboratory are briefly mentioned below as examples substantiating the validity of some of the questions that need to be answered.
In 11 patients with carcinoma of the colon, the in vivo uptake of labeled 5-fluorouracil (FU) and 5-fluorouridine (FUR) in tumor and adjacent normal tissue and the incorporation of label into RNA were measured in samples obtained at surgery. The precursors used were FU-2-^{14}C, FU-6-^{3}H, and FUR-2-^{14}C and were injected intravenously 30–60 min before surgery at a maximum radiolabel dose of 100 μCi per patient. The following observations were made:

1. With all three precursors, the variability in uptake into acid-soluble components was greater in tumor than in normal tissue;
2 With FUR, this uptake was greater in tumor than in normal tissue in two patients; it was the reverse in one and was low and not significantly different in three;
3. With FU, regardless of label, the uptake was greater in tumor than in normal tissue in three patients and was the reverse in one;
4. In four patients, incorporation of label into RNA was greater in tumor than in normal tissue, in two it was the converse, and in five it was insignificant in either tissue; in general the trends in uptake and incorporation were in parallel;
5. In no case could the variability among patients be ascribed to major differences in the time elapsing between the injection of the labeled precursor and the processing of the sample.

These results, although very preliminary indeed, are consistent with those previously obtained by others [4, 5] and allow four conclusions to be reasonably reached at this time:
1. There is a wide quantitative variability among patients in the way F-pyrimidines are handled in colon tumor and normal colonic mucosa;
2. In some patients uptake and incorporation were greater in tumor than in normal mucosa, consistent with potential selectivity of action against tumor; in some other patients the relationships were in the opposite direction or no significant uptake was noted, both findings being a priori inconsistent with potential selectivity of action against tumor;
3. It is essential that this type of information be correlated with clinical response to F-pyrimidines before its practical usefulness can be assessed and that it be compared with accumulation of FUdMP and inhibition of thymidylate synthetase (TMP-S);
4. It seems that measurements of possible determinants of F-pyrimidines action in target cells are indeed warranted and that identification of additional determinants is needed before a final selection of a set of useful measurements can be made.

In four patients, one with malignant melanoma, one with malignant fibrous histiocytoma, and two with sarcoma (one fibrosarcoma and one leiomysarcoma), a pyrimidine salvage enzyme profile diversity was noted. Because of the small number of patients examined so far, only the most salient observations can be tentatively mentioned at this time for the sake of discussion. There was clear evidence of variability among patients in the activities of thymidylate kinase (TMP-K), deoxycytidylate kinase (dCMP-K), thymidine kinase (TK), and uridine kinase (UK); in general TMP-K, dCMP-K, and UK seem to vary in concert whereas the pattern exhibited by TK is not yet definable. TMP-S activity was undetectable in lung and in the four tumors studied. In contrast, this enzyme had good activity in cells from five patients with AML. It is of interest in this respect that, in measuring TMP-S in different tissue culture cell lines, good activity was found in two lines derived from acute lymphoblastic leukemia but none was detected in three lines from melanoma. Should it be confirmed that TMP-S activity is unusually low or undetectable in cells from certain solid tumor, this finding would provide an obviously important basis for the design of chemotherapy, perhaps utilizing inhibitors of salvage pyrimidine pathways in preference to inhibitors of the de novo pathway.
Experiments were conducted in mice implanted subcutaneously with Lewis lung carcinoma, which develop lung metastasis with 7–10 days from transplantation. In initial experiments, comparisons were made between primary tumor and three different lung metastasis of comparable size, without at this time any measurements of cell kinetics. Again TMP-S

activity was undetectable; deoxycytosine kinase was low in primary tumor and undetectable in the metastasis; TMP-K was twice as high in primary tumor as compared to the metastasis; TK and deoxycytidylate deaminase were lower in primary tumor than in the metastasis; dCMP-K was similar in primary tumor and in one of the metastasis, but it was about two fold lower in the second metastasis and 13-fold lower in the third one. Thus, these results confirm that TMP-S is not detectable in certain tumors and indicate that differences in the activity of certain enzymes may occur not only between primary tumor and metastasis but also among different metastasis originating from the same primary tumor. This biochemical diversity is not surprising per se in light of the information that has been acquired in recent years suggesting the occurrence of diversity in biologic patterns and markers within heterogeneous cell populations from leukemias as well as solid tumors.

Concluding Remarks

The question whether it is reasonable to assume that the technical difficulties in design and sampling intrinsic to studies of determinants of drug action in solid tumors may be overcome can only be posed at this time. Examples of biologic and biochemical diversity within tumor, like those mentioned above, suggest that the intrinsic heterogeneity of tumor cell populations may represent a serious obstacle for the approach considered in this discussion. Should it become reasonable, however, to minimize these obstacles, will it be possible to obtain primary tumor samples with adequate biochemical integrity that could, as such or after isolation of different cell subsets, provide adequate representation of both original tumor and potential metastasis. Should this degree of confidence on the adequacy of samples be reached and should the necessary cell suspension and separation procedures be developed, would it become possible to identify determinants of drug action that could be predictive of response based on single time point measurements on samples obtained essentially only at surgery?

Obviously, enormous difficulties need to be overcome in order to be able to obtain predictive indices of response in patients with solid tumors based on measurements of target cell determinants of drug action. A large number of observations have been reported in the literature indicating that single parameters are usually not adequate predictors of drug action and may at best predict resistance. This is now well-understood as it is recognized that the activity of a drug will depend on a multiplicity of factors; thus, only single parameters that are the consequence of a summation of various effects may have predictive value, provided that their discriminating power remains sufficient despite the dampening effect summations usually have on sensitivity. It is because of this type of consideration that the earlier frustrations derived from observations on such isolated parameters as the inhibition of a putative target enzyme or the uptake of a drug may now find an explanation.

In this discussion, an attempt has been made to focus on the need for systematic studies of the multiple integrated biochemical pharmacologic determinants of drug action that may be identified in target cells and may aid in the design of adjuvant or secondary treatment of patients with solid tumor. It is obvious that these parameters should be further integrated with systemic pharmacokinetic and drug biotransformation measurements. Only after correlations between the different sets of determinants and the response of the patients are drawn will it become possible to achieve a reasonable selection of the ultimate parameters to be measured for each drug. Several of the basic difficulties to be met in applying the approaches discussed to the design of adjuvant treatments of patients with solid tumors have been alluded to and should under no circumstance be minimized. However, only by aggressively pursuing careful investigations aimed at answering some of the basic questions raised in this discussion will it become possible to conclude whether the approach considered herein only represents a wishful working hypothesis based on theoretical arguments or a clinical reality based on irrefutable results.

References

1. Chou, T.-C., Clarkson, B. D., Philips, F. S.: Metabolism of 1-β-D-Arabinosylcytosine in human leukemic cells. Cancer Res. *37,* 3561–3570 (1977)
2. Creaven, P. J., Rustum, Y. M., Slocum, H. K., Mittelman, A.: The clinical pharmacokinetics of 3-Deazauridine, a new antineoplastic agent. In: Current chemotherapy II, Proc. 10th Int. Congr. Chemotherapy. Siegenthaler, W., Luthy, R. (eds.), pp. 1208–1210. Washington, D.C.: Am. Soc. for Microbiology Pub. 1978
3. Mihich, E., et al.: Toxicological evaluation of new anticancer drugs. In: Current chemotherapy I, Proc. 10th Int. Congr. Chemotherapy. Siegenthaler, W., Luthy, R. (eds.), pp. 103–106. Washington, D.C.: Am. Soc. for Microbiology Pub. 1978
4. Mukherjee, K. L., Boohar, J., Wentland, D., Ansfield, F. J., Heidelberger, C.: Studies on fluorinated pyrimidines XVI. metabolism of 5-fluorouracil-2-^{14}C and 5-fluoro-2′-deoxyuridine-2-^{14}C in cancer patients. Cancer Res. *23,* 49–66 (1963)
5. Mukherjee, K. L., Curreri, A. R., Javid, M., Heidelberger, C.: Studies on fluorinated pyrimidines XVII. Tissue distribution of 5-fluorouracil-2-^{14}C and 5-fluoro-2′-deoxyuridine-2-^{14}C in cancer patients. Cancer Res. *23,* 67–77 (1963)
6. Rustum, Y. M.: Metabolism and intracellular retention of 1-β-D-arabinosyl cytosine as predictors of response of animal tumors. Cancer Res. *38,* 543–549 (1978)
7. Rustum, Y. M., Creaven, P. J., Slocum, H. K.: Biochemical and pharmacological studies of 3-deazauridine with L1210 cells susceptible and resistant to cytosine arabinoside. I: Current chemotherapy II, Proc. 10th Int. Congr. Chemotherapy. Siegenthaler, W., Luthy, R. (eds.), pp. 1118–1120. Washington, D.C.: 1978
8. Rustum, Y. M., Grindey, G. B., Hakala, M. T., Mihich, E.: Multifactorial cellular determinants of the action of antimetabolites. In: Advances in enzyme regulation. Weber, G. (ed.), pp. 281–295. New York, Oxford: Pergamon Press 1976
9. Rustum, Y. M., Preisler, H., Wrzosek, C., Wang, G., Rubenstein, J., Kelly, E.: Biochemical determinants of arabinosylcytosine (araC) action against acute myelocytic leukemia (AML) cells. Am. Soc. Clin. Oncol. *19,* 338 (1978)
10. Smith, J. F., Robins, A. B., Leese, C. L.: The metabolism of cytosine arabinoside as a predictive test for clinical response to the drug in acute myeloid leukemia. Eur. J. Cancer *12,* 567–573 (1976)

Post-Surgical Systematic Active Immunotherapy: Rational and Experimental Basis

G. Mathé, L. Olsson, I. Florentin, N. Kiger, S. Orbach-Arbouys, and J. I. Schulz

Those who accepted the preliminary results of postsurgical chemotherapy of minimal residual disease (MRD) with too much enthusiasm now feel deceived since the number of beneficial chemotherapy trials has not increased much and in addition the preliminary results in postmenopausal breast cancer are not any more significant [61] and in osteosarcoma they are markedly diminished [12, 14, 24]. This is a human but not a scientific deception for those who, realizing the mode of action of chemotherapy, have always stressed the fact that chemotherapy obeys first-order kinetics [65–67]: each cycle kills a number of logs of cells but this number re-increases during the intervals (Fig. 1a). Hence, the final loss depends on the number of logs of cells killed by each cycle, on the doubling time of the tumor, and on the interval (Fig. 1b) that makes the possibility of killing all cells highly improbable. Le Pecq et al. [30], studying the correlation between the number of cells killed and the dose of the oncostatic, were able by increasing the dose of the agent to increase this number to 99.99% but not to 99.999% (Fig. 1c). This might simply be due to the fact that a tumor cell population includes a

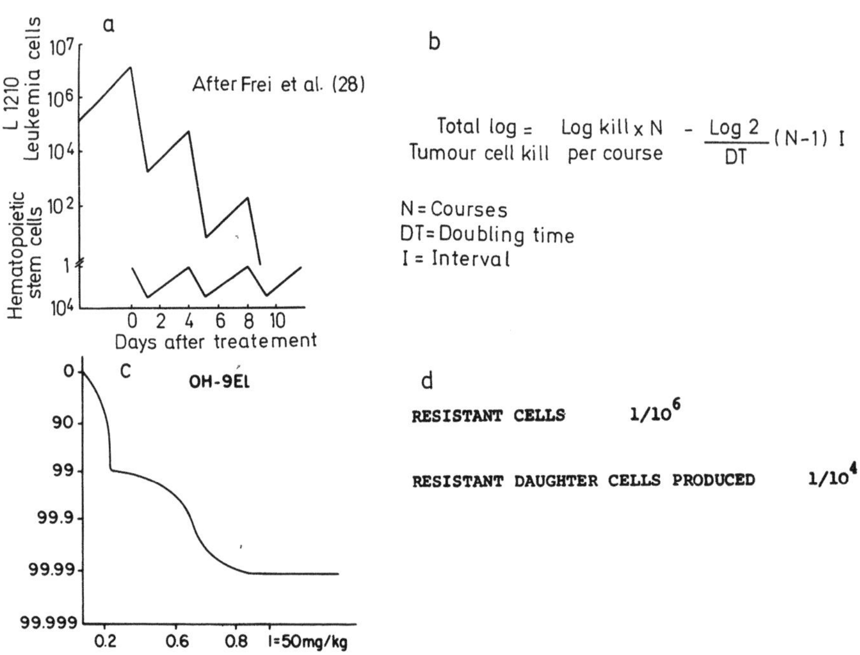

Fig. 1. a Chemotherapy obeys first-oder kinetics. **b** The effect of an intermittent chemotherapy depends on the number of cells killed in a cycle, the number of cycles, the intervals, and the doubling time. **c** Chemotherapy does not kill the last cell, which may be due to primary and secondary resistance **(d)**

priori 10^{-6} elements that are primarily resistant to chemotherapy and, after the application of the drug, 10^{-4} cells that are secondarily resistant [15]. We have been taking into consideration for many years the fact that chemotherapy does not kill "the last cell" [33] and we have attempted to achieve this by increasing the natural immune resistance to neoplastic elements, giving the name of *active immunotherapy* to the immune manipulation applied after the tumor was established [34, 39].

The result of adjuvant chemotherapy in osteosarcoma today is very much in favor of this proposed concept: the difference between the treated patients curve and the nontreated ones is large after 2 years and markedly diminishes after 4 years [24], which can only be explained by the fact that chemotherapy did not kill the last cells [33]. SALMON [62] established a remarkable curve for surgically treated breast cancer patients showing that all patients in whom 10^9 cells are left will relapse, and those carrying ten neoplastic cells have a 100% change to be cured (Fig. 2a).

This ten cell number seems to be of great importance, as it is precisely the mean inductive number of most murine grafted tumors, especially that of L1210 leukemia as we noticed 20 years ago (Fig. 2b). We have observed that ten cells of L1210 leukemia were needed to kill 50% of normal mice, while only one cell was necessary for obtaining the same mortality in immunodepressed animals, in which this natural immune resistance is decreased.

This observation led us to search for ways to augment this number in immunoprophylactic

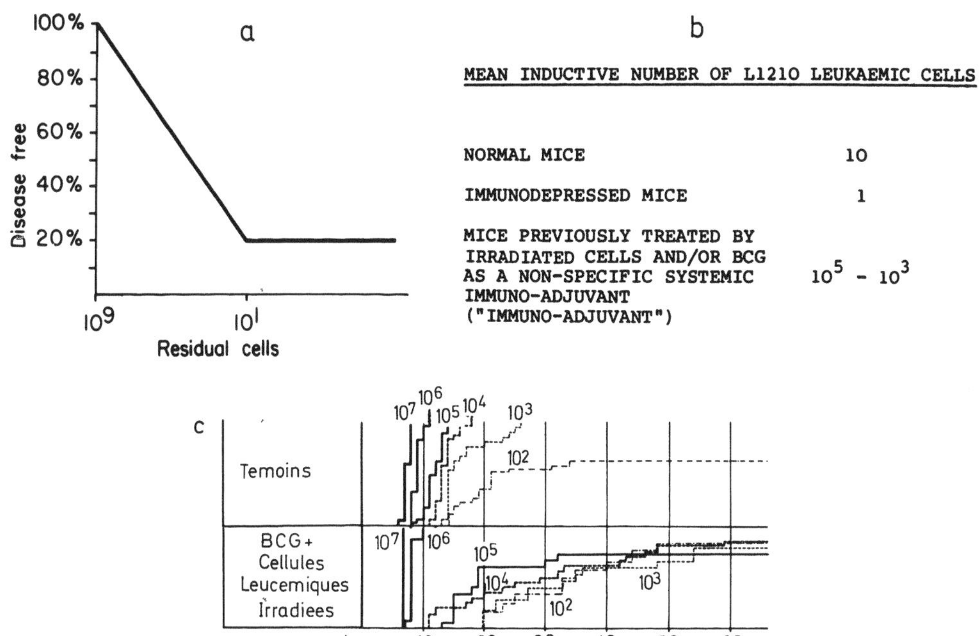

Fig. 2. a According to Salmon's (18) calculation, postsurgical minimal residual disease needs to be reduced to ten cells by chemotherapy to achieve 100% cure. **b** This number corresponds to the mean inductive number of L1210 leukemia in mice; it can be increased to 10^5 in an immunoprophylactic experiment employing BCG and a specific vaccine made of irradiated tumor cells. **c** It is also this number, 10^5 cells, that immunotherapy, i.e., immunomanipulation applied *after* the tumor is established, can eradicate

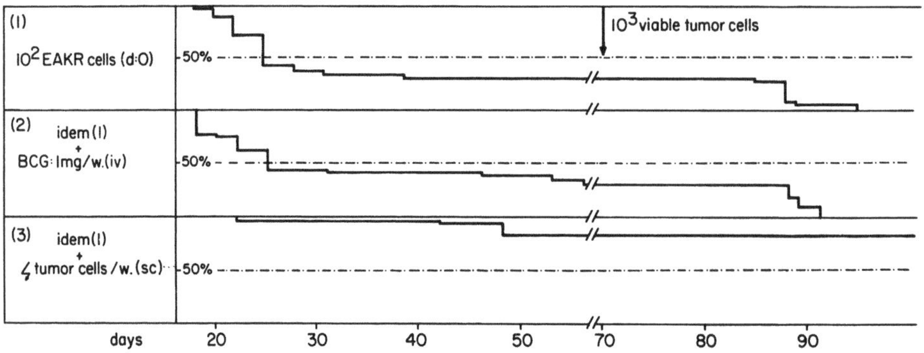

Fig. 3. Attempt at active systemic immunotherapy of EAkR murine leukemia inoculated with only 10^2 tumor cells, either with BCG alone (not effective) or with irradiated tumor cells alone (effective)

Table 1. Antitumoral effect of doses of irradiated tumor cells injected SC every week with start at day + 1 after tumor cell inoculation and given maximally eight times

Treatment	No. of tumor cells inoculated	Mean survival time of dying mice in days (range)	Non-tumor-bearing mice > 90 days after tumor inoculation (%)	Statistics[a]
None (controls)	10^2	28.0±1.8 (21–34)	10	–
	10^3	25.5±2.0 (20–29)	5	–
	10^5	16.8±1.6 (13–19)	0	–
	10^6	14.7±1.4 (12–16)	0	–
10^5 irradiated tumor cells injected SC per week start day + 1	10^2	35.2±3.8 (27–42)	10	N.S.
	10^3	32.0±3.6 (28–37)	5	N.S.
	10^5	15.8±2.0 (12–20)	0	N.S.
	10^6	15.0±1.6 (12–19)	0	N.S.
10^7 irradiated tumor cells injected SC per week start day + 1	10^2	47.4±6.5 (36–61)	70	$P < 0.01$
	10^3	42.7±5.6 (33–54)	45	$P < 0.01$
	10^5	17.8±1.4 (14–22)	0	N.S.
	10^6	15.6±2.0 (11–20)	0	N.S.
10^9 irradiated tumor cells injected SC per week start day + 1	10^2	43.1±7.0 (34–62)	65	$P < 0.01$
	10^3	46.4±4.1 (37–55)	50	$P < 0.01$
	10^5	16.3±1.9 (13–22)	0	N.S.
	10^6	14.6±1.1 (12–17)	0	N.S.
10^9 irradiated normal lymphoid cell injected SC per week start day + 1	10^2	25.0±2.5 (16–31)	10	N.S.
	10^3	22.6±2.0 (17–28)	0	N.S.
	10^5	15.3±1.7 (13–21)	0	N.S.
	10^6	14.3±2.2 (12–21)	0	N.S.

[a] Statistics have been performed with Wilcoxons' nonparametric test comparing survival of all control mice with the survival of the various immune-stimulated groups.

experiments where we succeeded in increasing it to 10^5 cells. We have treated L1210 leukemia [34, 39] and other neoplasias [37] with the same immunomanipulation (immunotherapy) after their establishment and were able to cure the animals carrying $\leqslant 10^5$ leukemic cells (Fig. 2c) [34].

We conducted our first trial of active immunotherapy in man in patients with acute lymphoid leukemia because in 1962 it was one of the rare diseases in which we were able to maintain a long remission with chemotherapy, and hence we thought that we might be able to reduce the number of postchemotherapy residual leukemia cells to a number accessible to active immunotherapy [40]. This randomized trial, in which seven of 20 patients in the immunotherapy branch are still in remission 16 years later versus 0 in the control group, induced, despite criticism to which we responded [46], many clinical trials on active immunotherapy. Some were in favor of our conclusion [11, 48] while others could not confirm it [70]. Since the same phenomenon has occurred with trials concerning other diseases [37, 70], one of the objects of this paper will be to try to explain the coexistence of negative and positive trials and to evaluate the factors of immunotherapy application that determine the types of results obtained.

In the first experiment on L1210 leukemia [34], we used cells as *specific immunotherapy* and/or BCG as *nonspecific immunotherapy*. We had shown in another experiment [39] that this combination was superior to the use of cells of BCG as single agents only. But this does not allow us to conclude that cells or adjuvant alone could not be, in some circumstances, sufficient to exert a significant action. As a matter of fact, we showed that, when the inoculated neoplastic cell population was very small (10^2) in the case of EAkR leukemia, irradiated cells alone were able to cure the animals that later resisted the challenge with the same tumor (Fig. 3) [28]. In man the most interesting trial using cells only (treated by

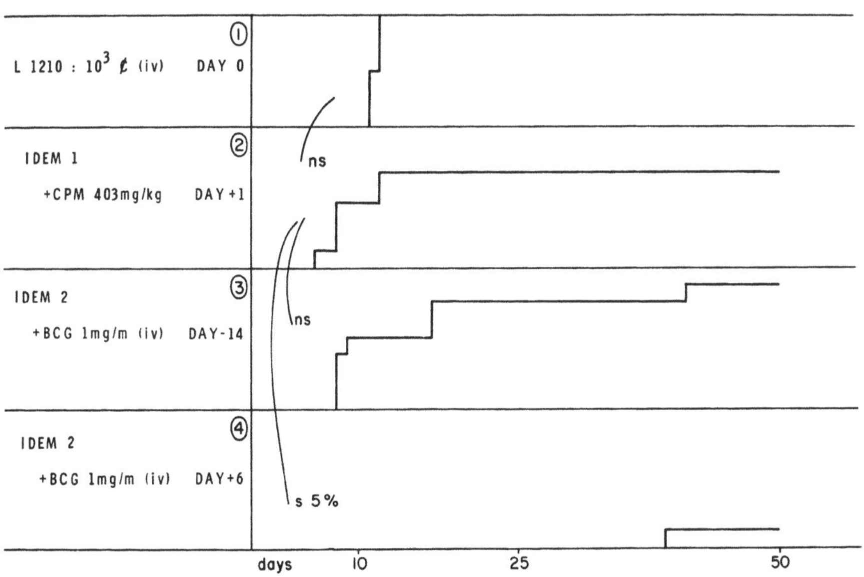

Fig. 4. Immunotherapeutic effect of BCG given 5 days after the injection of 403 mg/kg cyclophosphamide and its protective effect against early bone marrow (and lymphoid?) toxicity

neuraminidase) is that of acute myeloid leukemia conducted by BEKESI and HOLLAND [4] in which the benefit due to this specific immunotherapy is impressive.

There are several critical factors determining the effect of specific immunotherapy, i.e., the dose factor (Table 1) [51], and there are other substances such as the solubilized cell antigens where differences such as the solubilized cell antigens where differences in their preparation may lead to the opposing results [32]. On the other hand, immunity adjuvant alone may also be efficient as demonstrated with BCG applied after cell reduction by chemotherapy in L1210 leukemia (Fig. 4) [44]. Here also, there are factors that determine the effect of BCG, such as the preparation used [only the living Pasteur BCG is efficient in our screening: 42], and the route used [only the IV, the scarification, and heaf-gun administrations are efficient in our mice experiments: 31].

BCG can also be applied regionally, between the tumor and the lymph nodes, before surgery in the case of EAkR lymphosarcoma [9] and B16 melanoma [10] (regional active immunotherapy). BCG alone has been significantly effective in some human nonsolid tumors such as lymphosarcomas [7, 19]. Other trials have been negative [70], and it is of interest to consider not only the preparations and the route of administration used in each trial but other factors as well.

The dose of BCG might be the most important factor, as shown in our experiment in EAkR leukemia. There is an optimal dose, below which the effect is insignificant and over which it is

Table 2. Antitumoral effect of various doses of BCG injected IV every week with start at day + 1 after tumor cell inoculation and given maximally eight times

Treatment	No. of tumor cells inoculated	Mean survival time of dying mice in days (range)	Non-tumor-bearing mice > 90 days after tumor inoculation (%)	Statistics[a]
None	10^2	26.8±2.3 (19–32)	15	–
(controls)	10^3	23.1±1.9 (18–32)	5	–
	10^5	16.5±2.0 (12–20)	0	–
	10^6	15.3±1.6 (12–18)	0	–
1.4 × 10^6 viable	10^2	25.1±2.9 (18–31)	20	N.S.
units BCG IV	10^3	24.0±1.8 (19–30)	5	N.S.
per week	10^5	15.6±2.1 (11–19)	0	N.S.
start day + 1	10^6	14.9±1.7 (11–18)	0	N.S.
7 × 10^6 viable	10^2	32.3±4.7 (26–41)	45	$P < 0.01$
units BCG IV	10^3	29.3±3.6 (24–36)	35	$P < 0.01$
per week	10^5	17.8±1.9 (13–21)	25	$P < 0.01$
start day + 1	10^6	14.9±2.0 (11–19)	0	N.S.
21 × 10^6 viable	10^2	22.5±1.3 (17–25)	0	$P < 0.01$
units BCG IV	10^3	20.3±1.8 (15–24)	0	$P < 0.01$
per week	10^5	14.1±2.0 (11–18)	0	N.S.
start day + 1	10^6	14.2±2.3 (10–18)	0	N.S.

[a] Statistics have been performed with Wilcoxons' nonparametric test comparing survival of all mice in the control group with the survival of the various immune-stimulated groups.

also diminished (Table 2) [51]. We described the dose-effect correlation on the hemolytic plaque forming test in 1975: while a dose of 1 mg of BCG per mouse increased the response, 0.2 mg and 3 mg per mouse did not affect it and 10 mg decreased it (Table 3) [36]. We presume that doses smaller than the optimal one are insufficient to induce the septicemia shown necessary by KHALIL et al. [26] for an optimal action on murine leukemia, and we used in man a modality of application shown in Table 4 that adapts the dose to the immune status of the patients.

The problem of immunosuppression due to the dose higher than the optimal one was totally obscure we demonstrated with GEFFARD et al. [16] that it was due to the stimulation of suppressor cells by such doses (Table 5). This problem arises during the chronic as well as after single or short-term administration (Table 6) [27]. The next step was to try to eliminate suppressor cells (Fig. 5) by chemotherapy. We have demonstrated [52] that they could be destroyed with methotrexate (Table 7), while POLACK and TURK showed that they could be killed by cyclophosphamide [55].

There are in fact other reasons brought out by experimental data for alternating chemotherapy and immunotherapy: (a) chemotherapy is known to work mainly on cells in the cycle, while we showed with Olsson that immunotherapy mainly works on cells on G0 or in Gl phases (Fig. 6) [50]; (b) chemotherapy may not be efficient in immunodepressed animals (Fig. 7) [47] and some forms are immunodepressive [8]; hence, it is reasonable to attempt to restore immunity between chemotherapy cycles; (c) BCG stimulates hematorestoration after chemo-

Table 3. Influence of the dose of fresh living BCG (injected IV 14 days before antigen) on the humoral response of mice sheep red blood cells (Jerne test)

Dose (mg)	Index of stimulation	
10	$I^a = 0.06$ ↘	$S^b > 1\%$
5	$I = 1.3$	N.S.
1	$I = 4.01$ ↗	$S > 2\%$
0.5	$I = 4.01$ ↗	$S > 1\%$
0.1	$I = 1.64$	N.S.
Control	$I = 1$	

[a] $\frac{\text{Mean No. of PFC/spleen of experimental mice}}{\text{Mean No. of PFC/spleen of controls}}$.

[b] Student Fisher test. S, significant; N.S., not significant.

Table 4. Modality of BCG application

Delayed hypersensibility + one dose of 75 mg on one scarified area/week
Delayed hypersensibility + four doses of 75 mg on four scarified areas/week
If temperature < 38° C, the application is repeated the following day

Table 5. Mixed lymphocyte reaction between C57B1/6 normal or BCG-treated spleen cells and irradiated DBA/2 spleen cells

Dose of BCG injected to C57B1/6	CPM in cultures with irradiated C57B1/6 spleen cells	CPM in cultures with irradiated DBA/2 spleen cells
Day 7		
0 mg	3,486	9,944
1.5 mg	3.446	12,097
3.0 mg	3,554	6,181

Percent spleen 125 IUDR uptake in lethaly BFD_1 hybrids 4 days after C57B1/6 spleen cell injection

Treatment of donors	Treatment of recipients	
	None	Cycloheximide
No treatment BCG day 7	0.22	0.34
0.75 mg	0.19	0.32
1.5 mg	0.19	0.82
3.0 mg	0.30	0.66

Table 6. Effect of acute versus chronic administration of BCG on immune responses in mice

Immune responses		BCG treatment[a]					
		Control	0.2 mg 1 ×	0.2 mg 5 ×	1 mg 1 ×	1 mg 5 ×	5 mg 1 ×
Plaque-forming cell responses	TNP–POL	+	+	++	++++	+++	+++
	TNP–KLH	+	++	+++	++++	++	++++
Peritoneal macrophage cytostatic activity		–	+	+++	+++	+++	+++
Mitogen responsiveness	T cell mitogen	+++	++	+	±	–	–
	B cell mitogen	++	++	+++	+++	++	++
Suppressor cells	Macrophage	–	±	+	+	+	+
	T cells	–	–	±	–	+±	++

[a] Schedule of IV BCG treatment.

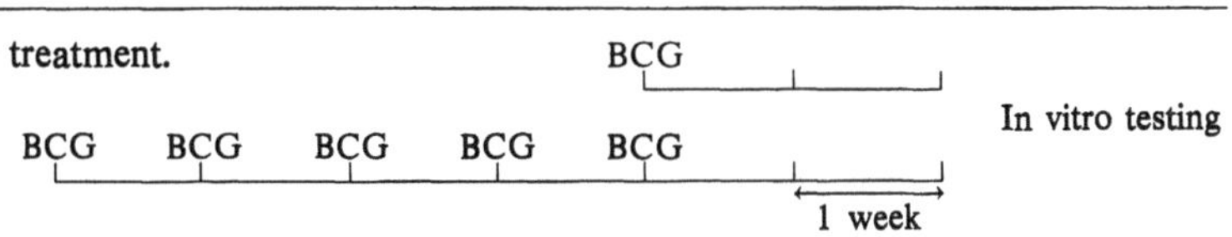

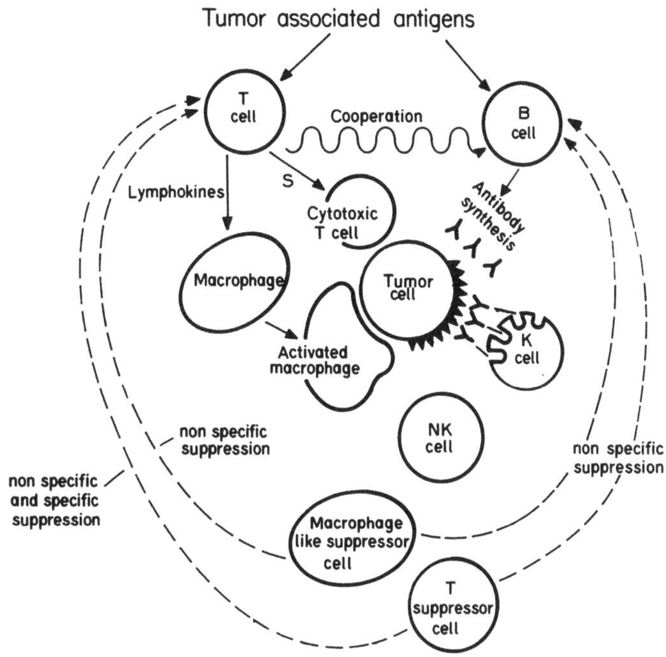

Fig. 5. A simplistic scheme depicting the process of natural resistance against tumors and its modulation by immunotherapy

therapy (Fig. 8) [35] and may shorten the intervals between two chemotherapy cycles.

Interspersion of BCG immunotherapy and of chemotherapy in several trials concerning acute myeloid leukemia has been significantly superior to chemotherapy alone [18, 57, 58, 71, 72, 75]. But not all trials of chemotherapy-immunotherapy interspersion gave a significant

Table 7. Possible effect of chemotherapy on suppressor cells PHA responsiveness of lymphoid cells after methotrexate injection

	5×10^5 Cells cultivated	
	Alone	With PHA
Controls	549 ± 196	13,408 ± 710
Methotrexate day 5	2,799 ± 531	27,246 ± 2,559
BCG 3 mg day 14	5,588 ± 722	7,831 ± 987
BCG 3 mg day 14 Methotrexate day 5	3,855 ± 45	20,052 ± 1,672

Enhancemant of the PHA reactivity (measured by the ^{3}H-thymidine incorporation in culture) of spleen cells from mice injected 5 days before the test with 0.5 mg methotrexate. The suppressed response of cells from BCG-injected animals is enhanced as much as the normal one.

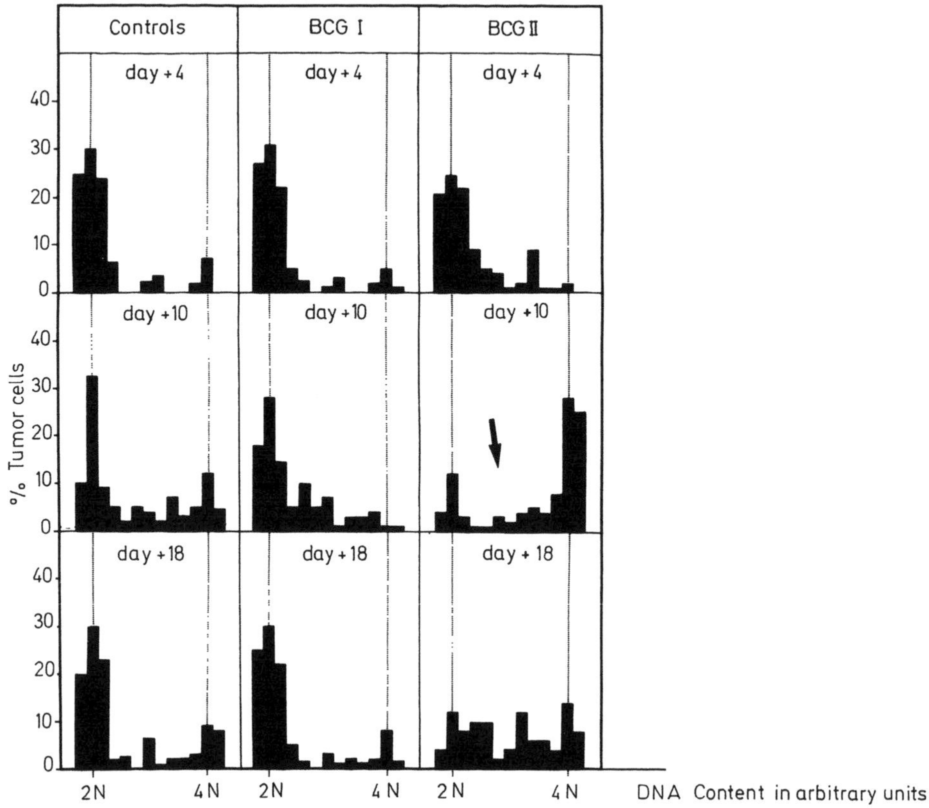

Fig. 6. Percentage distribution of ascitic tumor cells as a function of single-cell DNA content at various times after inoculation IP of 10^5 tumor cells. *2N* indicates the mean DNA content of Gl cells and *4N* the mean DNA content of mitoses (and G2 phase cells). Each value is the mean of 3—5 times. BCG I, BCG-treated mice with tumor load and tumor cell mitotic activity no different from controls; BCG II, BCG-treated mice with a lower tumor cell number and a higher tumor cell mitotic activity than controls

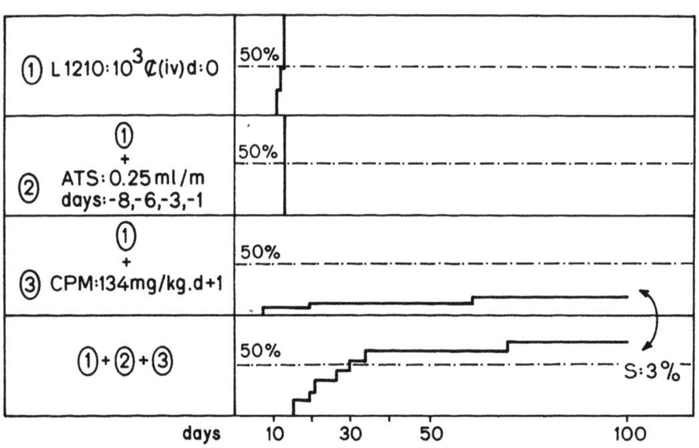

Fig. 7. Effect of antithymocyte serum-induced immunodepression on the oncostatic power of cyclophosphamide chemotherapy. Results are expressed in percentage of cumulative mortality of leukemia-bearing mice. Statistical significance is calculated by Wilcoxon's nonparametric test

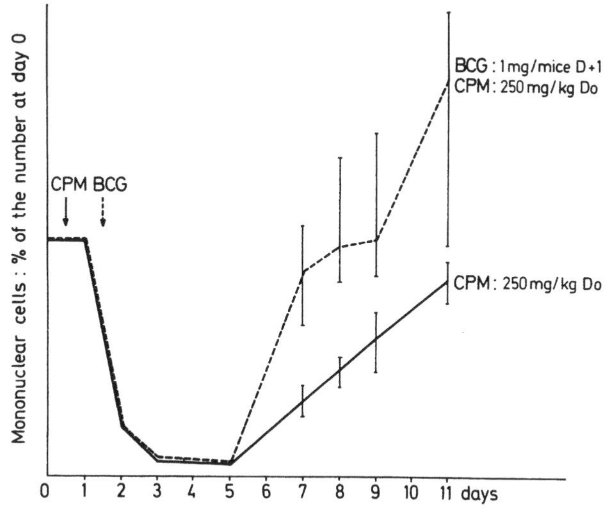

Fig. 8. Effect of BCG on lymphoid stem cells: the restoration of blood lymphocyte number after cyclophosphamide aplasia is faster when BCG is administered 1 day after cytostatics

benefit [70]. Moreover, by experimentally applying several cycles of interspersed cyclophosphamide and of BCG in L1210 leukemia, we obtained a result that was inferior compared to the use of one cycle alone consisting of cyclophosphamide (CPM) followed by BCG [45]. As the sequence cyclophosphamide → BCG is more efficient than CPM or BCG alone, we questioned whether the sequence BCG → CMP might not be the cause for this deterioration, which was subsequently demonstrated to be the case (Fig. 9) [44]. We have shown in an allogeneic skin graft experiment that such a sequence can be strongly immunosuppressive, and we explained it by the fact that BCG pushes lymphocytes into the cycle, which makes them more sensitive to the cytostatic effect of CPM, a phase-dependent agent [43]. But although this is true for CPM it is not valid for some sugar derivatives of nitrosoureas [22]. The combination of RFNCU with BCG, even in the sequence BCG → RFCNU, is more efficient than the cytostatic alone or BCG alone (Fig. 10) [5]. Thus, the choice of cytostatic in chemotherapy-immunotherapy interspersion is the determinant. The choice of the immunity adjuvant may also be crucial.

As seen in Table 8, BCG acts on all populations of cells with a role in immune reactions, including suppressor cells.

Among other adjuvants of the second generation, Corynebacterium *parvum* is one of the most active, but it exerts inhibition of some T cell reactions [64] probably via a stimulating action on suppressor cells. This could explain why this adjuvant has given the only randomized trial in which a deteriorating effect has been significant [13]. Among interesting adjuvants that have been the object of much work are the polynucleotides, poly I:poly C [41] and poly A:poly U [54], which are immunostimulants of T-lymphocytes and of macrophages, the latter probably via T-lymphocytes, and under some conditions via induction of interferon, which is in itself an adjuvant stimulating macrophages (Table 8) [63]. Several polysaccharides such as krestin [69] may also act as adjuvants, stimulating mainly macrophages. One of the most interesting agents is levamisole. For years, we were unable to detect any effect, contrary to Renoux and Renoux [59], probably because we were working with 3-month-old mice. Recently, searching for agents able to restore old mice depleted of T cells, we

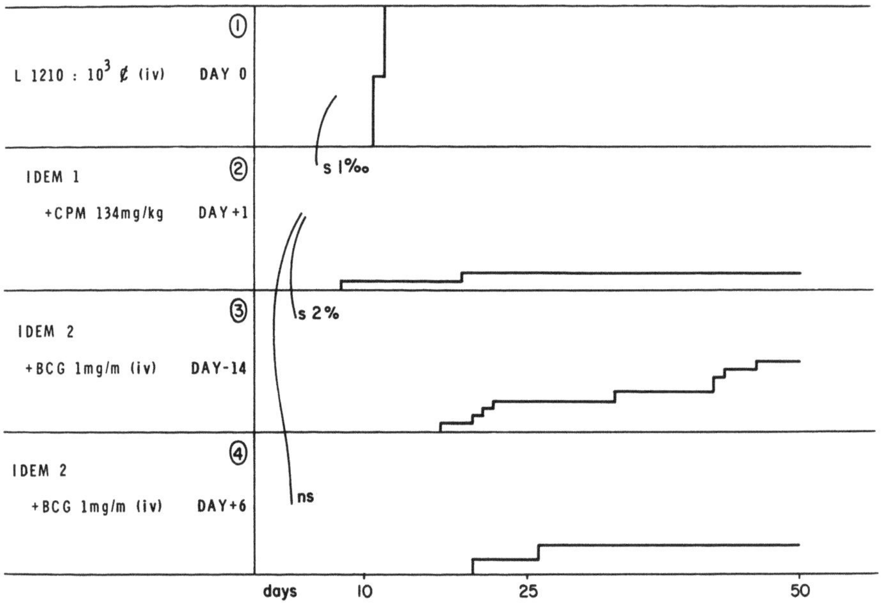

Fig. 9. Survival of mice carrying L1210 leukemia. Deterioration by BCG given before 134 mg/kg cyclophosphamide on its antileukemic effect

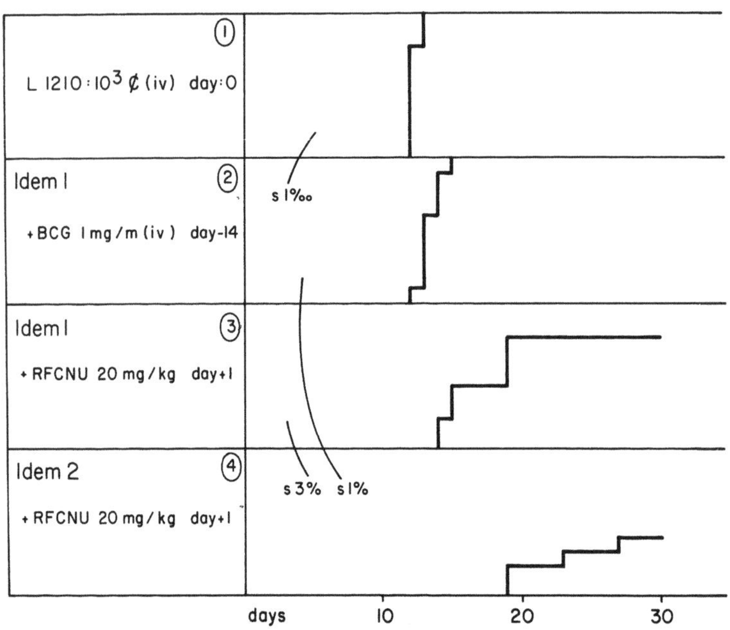

Fig. 10. The sequence BCG-RFCNU (a nonimmunosuppressive drug at the dose used) enhances the effect of both agents (contrary to the sequence of BCG-cyclophosphamide an immunosuppressive agent)

Table 8. Main immunologic actions of BCG and of the second generation of immunity adjuvants[a]

Immunologic parameters	BCG	C. parvum	Polynucleotides		Polysaccharides
			Poly I:C	Poly A:U	(ex: krestin)
Delayed hypersensitivity	↗	↘			↗
Humoral responses	↗	↗	↗	↗	↗
Suppressor cells	↗ ↗	↗ ↗ ↗	→	→	?
K cells	↗	↗	→	↘	?
Macrophage activation	↗ ↗	↗ ↗	↗	↗	↗ ↗
Interferon induction			+	?	?

[a] Those in italics are the object of trials presented in this meeting.

Table 9. Effect of acute and chronic administration of levamisole to 12-month-old mice

Immune response tested (at the age of 18 months)		Acute treatment[a]	Chronic treatment[a]
Spleen cell response to	PHA	1.24[b] →	0.43 ↘
	DS	1.00 →	1.41 ↗
T cell (nylon nonadherent cell) response to	PHA	0.85 →	0.83 →
Test for suppressor cell detection, mitogen response of normal spleen cells cocultivated with			
Unfractionated levamisole-treated cells	PHA	1.43 ↗ (−)	0.67 ↘ (+)
	DS	0.91 → (−)	1.33 ↗ (−)
Nylon nonadherent levamisole-treated cells	PHA	0.86 → (−)	1.04 → (−)
	DS	0.87 → (−)	1.34 ↗ (−)
Macrophage cytostatic activity in vitro, % inhibition of tumor cell proliferation		0%	Not tested
Antibody response to SRBC		1.54 ↗	2.57 ↗

[a] The chronic treatment consisted in weekly IP injections of 75 μg levamisole over a period of 6 months. The acute treatment consisted in a single IP injection of 75 μg levamisole at the same time as the last injection of the chronic treatment. Tests were performed 15 days after the last injection.

[b] $\frac{\text{Response of levamisole-treated mice;}}{\text{Response of control mice}}$.

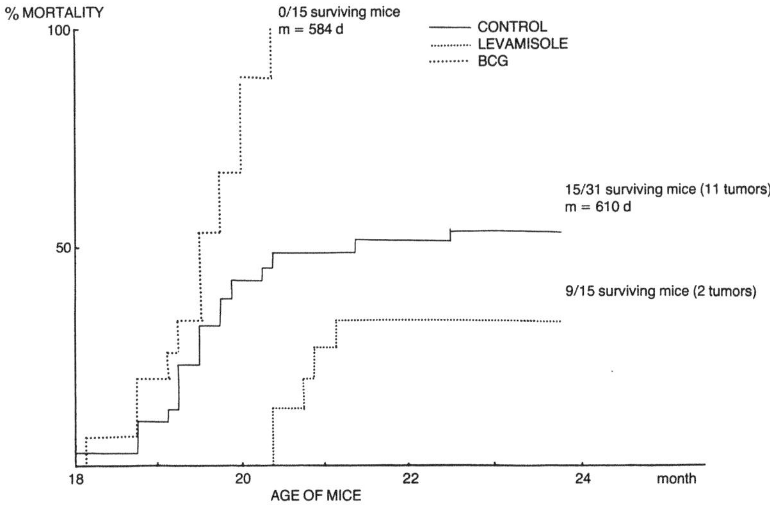

Fig. 11. Incidence of spontaneous tumors that appeared in three groups of (DBA/2 × C57Bl10) Fl aged mice submitted either to levamisole, BCG, or not treated

observed an immunorestorative effect of levamisole (Table 9) [6] and noticed that mice given this adjuvant developed less spontaneous tumors than nontreated animals, while BCG applied to another group not only did not restore the immune functions, but increased the incidence of spontaneous tumors (Fig. 11) [6]. The effect of levamisole was demonstrated in human acute lymphoid leukemia by PAVLOVSKY et al. [54]. In conclusion:

a) Active immunotherapy has now been the object of a reasonable number of trials in a variety of tumors, and the beneficial effect shown is significant not only in leukemias and lymphosarcomas quoted in this paper but also in solid tumors (Table 10) [1, 2, 17, 20, 21, 23, 25, 38, 49, 53, 56, 60, 68, 73, 74];

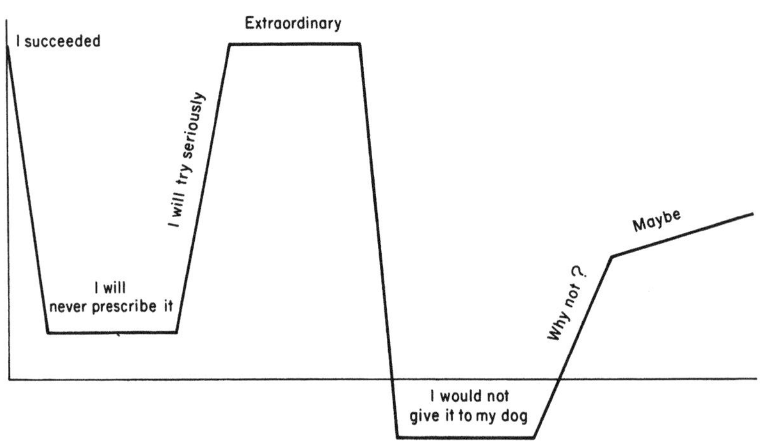

Fig. 12. The natural evolution of a new therapeutic means: immunotherapy seems to follow these kinetics

Table 10. Minimal residual disease immunotherapy randomized trials with presently significant favorable results

	Immunotherapy alone				Immunotherapy + chemotherapy > chemotherapy			
	Cells + BCG	BCG	Levamisole	Krestin	BCG + cells	Cells or "purified" antigen	BCG	BCG and C. parvum
Acute lymphoid leukemia	Mathé et al. [15, 18] EORTC, H.W.P. [17]		Pavlovsky et al. [59]					
Lymphosarcoma		Hoerni et al. [29] Cabanillas et al. [30]						
Acute myeloid leukemia					Powles et al. [42] Uden et al. [46]	Bekesi and Holland [21]	Vogler et al. [72]	
Bronchus		Pouillart et al. [69] McKneally et al. [67]	Amery [62]			Stewart et al. [71]		
Melanoma		Ikonopisov [65] Kaufman et al. [66] Paterson et al. [68]	Gonzales and Spitler [63]				Kaufman et al. [66]	Jacquillat et al. [74]
Breast			Rojas et al. [70]					
Head and Neck			Wanebo et al. [73]					
Stomach				Taguchi [56]				
Ovary					Hudson et al. [64]		Alberts [61]	

b) We know at least two reasons for explaining BCG negative trials: not applying enough or administering too much of BCG, which induces suppressor cells;
c) The parameters that have been shown to determine the effect of BCG have to be studied for other adjuvants that have already given significant beneficial results;
d) This underlines clearly the need for valuable monitoring: at the present time only the increase of null cells has been found significant [3]. The demonstration of monocyte decrease might also be an important modification [3]; similarly suppressor cells were found in some conditions. [ORBACH ARBOYS, unpublished].

The second and third generations of adjuvants (the latter discussed in our paper at the end of this volume), the knowledge of factors determining their action, and the importance of the monitoring may now place active immunotherapy in the last portion of the "normal" curve depicting the kinetics of any new therapeutic weapon (Fig. 12).

References

1. Alberts, D. S.: Adjuvant immunotherapy with BCG of advanced ovarian cancer: a preliminary report. In: Adjuvant therapy of cancer. Salmon, S. E., Jones, S. E. (eds.), pp. 327–334. Amsterdam, Oxford, New York: North Holland 1977
2. Amery, W.: Final results of a multicenter placebo controlled levamisole study of resectable lung cancer. In: Immune modulation and control of neoplasia by adjuvant therapy. Chirigos, M. A. (ed.). Cancer Treat. Rep. (1978) (in press)
3. Belpomme, D., Joseph, R., Lelarge, N.: Increase null cells in patients submitted to long-term active immunotherapy. Cancer Immunol. Immunother. *1*, 113–114 (1976)
4. Bekesi, J. G., Holland, J. F.: Active immunotherapy in leukaemia with neuraminidase modified leukemic cells. In: Tactics and strategy in cancer treatment. Mathé, G. (ed.), pp. 78–89. Heidelberg, New York: Springer 1977
5. Bruley Rosset, M., Florentin, I., Kiger, N., Mathé, G.: Comparative experimental immunopharmacology of three nitrosoureas: RFCNU, RPCNU and chlororzotocin. (in preparation) (1978)
6. Bruley Rosset, M., Florentin, I., Kiger, N., Davigny, M., Mathé, G.: Comparisons of the effects of BCG and levamisole administration in young adult and aged mice. In: Immune modulation and control of neoplasia by adjuvant therapy. Chirigos, M. A. (ed.). Cancer Treat. Rep. (1978) (in press)
7. Cabanillas, F., Rodriguez, V., Bodey, G. P.: The impact of intensive chemotherapy on the duration of remission and survival of patients (PTS) with nodular malignant lymphomas (NML). Proc. Am. Soc. Clin. Oncol. *19*, Abs. C-16 (1978)
8. Clarysse, A., Kenis, Y., Mathé, G.: Cancer chemotherapy. Its role in the treatment strategy of hematologic malignancies and solid tumors. Heidelberg, New York: Springer 1976
9. Economides, F., Bruley Rosset, M., Mathé, G.: Effect of pre-surgical active BCG immunotherapies on murine EAkR lymphosarcoma. Biomedicine *25*, 372–375 (1976)
10. Economides, F., Bruley Rosset, M., Mathé, G.: Treatment of the B16 melanoma with tumorectomy combined or not with adenectomy, systemic or/and regional BCG immunotherapy. Med. Oncol. *3*, S34 (1977)
11. EORTC Hemopathies Working Party, presented by P. Strychmans: A randomized trial comparing immunotherapy and chemotherapy as maintenance treatment of acute lymphoblastic leukemia. 2nd International Symposium on Therapy of Acute Leukemias. Rome, December 1977. (Abs. p. 129)

12. EORTC Osteosarcoma Working Party Group, presented by C. Jasmin: A randomized trial of adjuvant chemotherapy in osteogenic osteosarcoma: comparison of the alternance of sequential administrations of high doses adriamycin, methotrexate and cyclophosphamide with a 6 months administration of high dose adriamycin followed by a low dose semi continuous chemotherapy. In: RRCR Vol. 68, pp. 28–32. Berlin, Heidelberg, New York: Springer 1979
13. Fortner, J. G.: Management of recurrent malignant melanoma. 3rd International Symposium on Oncology. Teheran, March 1978 (Abs. 21)
14. Fossati-Bellani, F., Gasparini, M., Bonadonna, G.: Adriamycin in the adjuvant treatment of operable osteosarcoma. In: RRCR Vol. 68, pp. 25–27. Berlin, Heidelberg, New York: Springer 1979
15. Frei, E. (III.), Jaffe, N., Skipper, H. E., Gero, M. G.: Adjuvant chemotherapy of osteogenic sarcoma. Progress and perspectives. In: Adjuvant therapy of cancer. Salmon, S. E., Jones, S. J. (eds.), pp. 49–64. Amsterdam: Elsevier North Holland Biomedical Press 1977
16. Geffard, M., Orbach Arbouys, S.: Enhancement of T-suppressor activity in mice by high doses of BCG. Cancer Immunol. Immunother. *1*, 41–43 (1976)
17. Gonzalez, R., Spitler, L.: Effect of levamisole as a surgical adjuvant therapy on malignant melanoma. In: Immune modulation and control of neoplasia by adjuvant therapy. Chirigos, M. A. (ed.) Cancer Treat. Rep. (1978) (in press)
18. Gutterman, J. U., Rodrigues, V., Mavligit, G., Burgess, M. A., Gehan, E., Hersh, E. M., McCredie, K. B., Reed, R., Smith, T., Bodey, G. P. (Jr.), Preireich, E. J.: Chemo-immunotherapy of adult acute leukaemia prolongation of remission in myeloblastic leukemia with BCG. Lancet *2*, 1405–1409 (1974)
19. Hoerni, B., Chauvergne, J., Hoerni-Simon, G., Durand, M., Brunet, R., Lagarde, C.: BCG in the immunotherapy of Hodgkin's disease and non-Hodgkin's lymphomas. Results of a controlled trial including 60 patients. Cancer Immunol. Immunother. *1*, 109–112 (1976)
20. Hudson, C. N., Levin, L., McHardy, J. E., Poulton, R. A., Curling, O. M., Crowther, M., English, P. E., Leighton, M.: Active specific immunotherapy for ovarian cancer. Lancet *2*, 877–878 (1976)
21. Ikonopisov, R. L.: The use of BCG in the combined treatment of malignant melanoma. Behring Inst. Mitt. *56*, 206–214 (1975)
22. Imbach, J. L., Montero, J. L., Moruzzi, A., Serrou, B., Chenu, E., Hayat, M., Mathé, G.: The oncostatic and immunosuppressive action of new nitrosourea derivatives containing sugar radicals. Biomedicine *23*, 410–413 (1975)
23. Jacquillat, C., Banzet, P., Civatte, J., Puissant, A., Cottenot, F., Israel, L., Berlaich, S., Chastaing, Cl., Maral, J.: Adjuvant chemotherapy or immunotherapy in the management of primary melanoma of level III, IV or V (in this volume)
24. Jaffe, N.: 3rd Annual meeting of the medical oncology society. Nice. 4–6 December 1977
25. Kaufman, S. D., Carey, R. W., Cosimi, A. B., Wood, W. C.: Randomized trial of adjuvant therapy of "high risk" primary malignant melanoma. Proc. Am. Soc. Clin. Oncol. *19*, 374 (1978) (Abs. C-271)
26. Khalil, A., Bourut, C., Halle Pannenko, O., Mathé, G., Rappaport, H.: Histologica reactions or the thymus spleen, liver and lymph-nodes to intravenous and subcutaneous BCG injections. Biomedicine *22*, 112–121 (1975)
27. Kiger, N., Bruley Rosset, M., Florentin, I., Schulz, J., Mathé, G.: Effect of acute versus chronic administration of BCG on immune responses in mice. (in preparation) (1978)
28. Kiger, N., Olsson, L., Florentin, I., Mathé, G.: Specific active immunotherapy of EAkR leukaemia (in preparation) (1978)
29. Lacour, F., Lacour, J., Spira, A.: Poly A-Poly U as an adjunct to surgery in the treatment of spontaneous murine mammary adenocarcinoma. In: Investigation and stimulation of immunity in cancer patients. Mathé, G., Weiner, R. (eds.), pp. 352–358. Heidelberg, New York: Springer 1974

30. Le Pecq, J. B., Dat-Xuong, N., Gosse, C., Paoletti, C.: A new antitumoral agent: 9 hydroxyellipticine. Possibility of a rational design of anticancerous drugs in the series of DNA intercalating drugs. Proc. Natl. Acad. Sci. USA *71*, 5078–5082 (1974)
31. Martin, M., Bourut, C., Halle Pannenko, O., Mathé, G.: Routes other than i.v. injection to mice for BCG administration in active immunotherapy of L1210 leukemia. Biomedicine *23*, 339–340 (1975)
32. Martyre, M. C., Weiner, R., Halle Pannenko, O.: The in vivo activity of soluble extract obtained from RC19 leukemia: the effect of the method of extraction. In: Investigation and stimulation of immunity in cancer patients. Mathé, G., Weiner, R. (eds.), pp. 405–407. Heidelberg, New York: Springer 1974
33. Mathé, G.: La dernière cellule. Presse Méd. *75*, 2591–2593 (1967)
34. Mathé, G.: Immunothérapie active de la leucémie L1210 appliquée aprés la greffe tumorale. Rev. Fr. Etudes. Clin. Biol. *13*, 881–883 (1968)
35. Mathé, G.: Prevention of chemotherapy complications: time toxicity, pharmacokinetic and logistic factors. In: Complications of cancer chemotherapy. Mathé, G., Oldman, R. K. (eds.). Berlin, Heidelberg, New York: Springer 1974
36. Mathé, G.: Side effects and possible harmful action of immunomanipulation. In: The prediction of chronic toxicity from short term studies. pp. 67–82. Amsterdam: Excerpta Medica 1975
37. Mathé, G.: Active immunotherapy of cancer. Immunoprophylaxis and immunorestoration. An introduction, 1st. ed. Berlin, Heidelberg, New York: Springer 1976
38. Mathé, G.: Is systemic active immunotherapy shifting from the middle age to a renaissance period? 1. The multiplication of randomized trials showing significant effect of active immunotherapy on residual minimal disease. Cancer Immunol. Immunother. (1978) (in press)
39. Mathé, G., Pouillart, P., Lapeyraque, F.: Active immunotherapy of L1210 leukaemia applied after the graft of tumour cells. Br. J. Cancer *23*, 814–824 (1969)
40. Mathé, G., Amiel, J. L., Schwarzenberg, L., Schneider, M., Cattan, A., Schlumberger, J. R., Hayat, M., De Vassal, F.: Active immunotherapy for acute lymphoblastic leukaemia. Lancet *1969 I*, 697–699
41. Mathé, G., Hayat, M., Sakouhi, M., Choay, J.: L'action immuno-adjuvante du poly I:C chez la souris et son application au traitement de le L1210. C.R. Acad. Sci. (Paris) *272*, 170–173 (1971)
42. Mathé, G., Halle Pannenko, O., Bourut, C.: BCG in cancer immunotherapy. II. Results obtained with various BCG preparations in a screenin study for systemic adjuvants applicable to cancer immunoprophylaxis or immunotherapy. Natl. Cancer Inst. Monogr. *39*, 107–112 (1973)
43. Mathé, G., Halle Pannenko, O., Bourut, C.: Potentiation of a cyclophosphamide induced immunodepression by the administration of BCG. Transplant. Proc. *6*, 431–433 (1974)
44. Mathé, G., Halle Pannenko, O., Bourut, C.: Immune manipulation by BCG administered before or after cyclophosphamide for chemoimmunotherapy of L1210 leukaemia. Eur. J. Cancer *10*, 661–665 (1974)
45. Mathé, G., Halle Pannenko, O., Bourut, C.: Interspersion of cyclophosphamide and BCG in the treatment of L1210 leukaemia and Lewis tumour. Eur. J. Cancer *13*, 1095–1098 (1977)
46. Mathé, G., Amiel, J. L., Schwarzenberg, L., Schneider, M., Cattan, A., Schlumberger, J. R., Hayat, M., De Vassal, F.: Follow-up of the first (1962) pilot study on active immunotherapy of acute lymphoid leukaemia: a critical discussion. Biomedicine *24*, 29–35 (1977)
47. Mathé, G., Halle Pannenko, O., Bourut, C.: Effectiveness of murine leukemia chemotherapy according to the immune state reconsideration of correlations between chemotherapy tumor cell killing and survival time. Cancer Immunol. Immunother. *2*, 139–141 (1977)
48. Mathé, G., De Vassal, F., Schwarzenberg, L., Delgado, M., Weiner, R., Gil, M. A., Pena-Angulo, J., Belpomme, D., Pouillart, P., Machover, D., Misset, J. L., Pico, J. L., Jasmin, C., Hayat, M., Schneider, M., Cattan, A., Amiel, J. L., Musset, M., Rosenfeld, C., Ribaud, P.: Preliminary results of three protocols for the treatment of acute lymphoid leukaemia of children: distinction of two groups of patients according to predictable prognosis. Med. Pediatr. Oncol. *4*, 17–27 (1978)

49. McKneally, M. F., Maver, C. H., Kausel, H. W.: Intrapleural BCG immunostimulation in lung cancer. Lancet *1*, 1003 (1977)
50. Olsson, L., Mathé, G.: A cytokinetic analysis of bacillus Calmette Guérin induced growth control of murine leukemia. Cancer Res. *37*, 1743–1749 (1977)
51. Olsson, L., Ebbessen, P., Kiger, N., Florentin, I., Mathé, G.: The antileukemic effect of systemic non-specific BCG immunostimulation with irradiated isogenic leukemic cells. Eur. J. Cancer *14*, 355–362 (1978)
52. Orbach Arbouys, S., Castes, M., Berardet, M.: Enhancement of immunological responses by methotrexate pretreatment as a result of an eventual elimination of suppressor cells. In: Experiental hematology to-day. Berlin, Heidelberg, New York: Baum Springer (in press) (1978)
53. Paterson, A. H. G., Watson, M., Williams, D., McPherson, T. A.: Bacille Calmette-Guerin (BCG) immunotherapy in stage I, Clark's level (CL) 3–5 malignant melanoma. Proc. Am. Soc. Clin. Oncol. *19*, 389 (1978) (Abst. C-332)
54. Pavlovsky, S., Garay, G., Giraud, C., Sackman, F., Hayes, A., Svarch, E.: Chemo-immunotherapy with levamisole (LMS) in acute lymphocytic leukemia (ALL). Proc. Am. Assoc. Cancer Res. *19*, 204 (1978) (Abs. 814)
55. Polak, L., Turk, J. L.: Reversal of immunological tolerance by cyclophosphamide through inhibition of suppressor cell activity. Nature *249*, 654–656 (1974)
56. Pouillart, P., Mathé, G., Palangie, T., Schwarzenberg, L., Huguenin, P., Morin, P., Gautier, M., Parrot, R.: Trial of BCG immunotherapy in the treatment of resectable squamous cell carcinoma on the bronchus (stage I and II). Cancer Immunol. Immunother. *1*, 271–273 (1973)
57. Powles, R. L., Crowther, D., Beteman, C. J. T., Beard, M. E. J., Mac Elwain, T. J., Russel, J., Lister, T. A., Whitehouse, J. M. A., Wrigley, P. F. M., Pike, M., Alexancer, P., Hamilton Fairley, G.: Immunotherapy for acute myelogenous leukaemia. Br. J. Cancer *28*, 365–376 (1973)
58. Reizenstein, P., Brenning, G., Engstedt, L., Franzen, S., Gahrton, G., Gullbring, B., Holm, G., Hocker, P., Hoglund, S., Hornstein, P., Jamenson, S., Killander, A., Killander, D., Klein, E., Lantz, B., Lidemalm, C., Lockner, D., Lonnqvist, B., Mellstedt, H., Palmblad, J., Pauli, C., Skarberg, K. O., Uden, A. M., Vanky, F., Wadman, B.: Effect of immunotherapy on survival and remission duration in acute, non-lymphatic leukaemia. In: Immunotherapy of cancer: present status of trials in man. Terry, W. D., Windhorst, D. (eds.), pp. 329–339. New York: Raven Press 1978
59. Renoux, G., Renoux, M.: Levamisole inhibits and cures a solid malignant tumour and its pulmonary metastases in mice. Nature New Biol. *240*, 217–218 (1972)
60. Rojas, A. F., Feierstein, J. N., Glait, H. M., Olivari, A. J.: Levamisole action in breast cancer stage III. In: Immunotherapy of cancer: present status of trial in man. Terry, W. D., Windhorst, D. (eds.), pp. 635–645. New York: Raven Press 1978
61. Rossi, A., Valagussa, P., Bonadonna, G.: Combined modality management of operable breast cancer (in this volume)
62. Salmon, S. E.: Kinetic rationale for adjuvant chemotherapy of cancer. In: Adjuvant therapy of cancer. Salmon, S. E., Jones, S. J. (eds.), pp. 15–27. Amsterdam, Elsevier North Holland Biomedical Press 1977
63. Schultz, R. M., Chirigos, M. A., Pavlidis, N., Stylos, W.: Cytotoxic activity of interferon treated macrophages studied by various inhibitors. In: Immune modulation and control of neoplasia by adjuvant therapy. Chirigos, M. A. (ed.). Cancer Treat. Rep. (1978) (in press)
64. Scott, M. T.: Depression of delayed-type hypersensitivity by Corynebacterium parvum: mandatory role of the spleen. Cell. Immunol. *13*, 251–263 (1974)
65. Skipper, H. E., Schabel, F. M., Wilcox, W. S.: Experimental evaluation of potential anticancer agents. XIII. On the criteria and kinetics associated with "curability" of experimental leukemia. Cancer Chemother. Rep. *35*, 1–111 (1964)
66. Skipper, H. E., Schabel, F. M., Wilcox, W. S.: Experimental evaluation of potential anticancer agents. XIV. Further study of certain basic concepts underlying chemotherapy of leukemia. Cancer Chemother. Rep. *45*, 5–28 (1966)

67. Skipper, H. E., Schabel, F. M., Wilcox, W. S.: Experimental evaluation of potential anticancer agents. XXI. Schedulling of arabinosylcytosine to take advantage of its S-phase specificity against leukaemic cells. Cancer Chemother. Rep. *51*, 125–165 (1967)
68. Stewart, T. H. M., Hollinshead, A. C., Harris, J. E., Raman, S., Belanger, R., Crepeau, A., Crook, A. F., Hirte, W. E., Hooper, D., Klaassen, D, J., Rapp, E. F., Sachs, H. J.: Survival study of immunochemotherapy in lung cancer. In: Immunotherapy of cancer: present status of trial in man. Terry, W. D., Windhorst, D. (eds.), pp. 203–216. New York: Raven Press 1978
69. Taguchi, T.: Experimental and clinical studies on krestin. In: Immune modulation and control neoplasia of neoplasia by adjuvant therapy. Chirigos, M. A. (ed.). Cancer Treat. Rep. (1978) (in press)
70. Terry, W. D., Windhorst, D. (ed.): Immunotherapy of cancer: present status of trials in man. New York: Raven Press 1978
71. Udem, A. M., Lindemalm, C., Pauli, C., Vanky, F., Reizenstein, P.: Effects of immunotherapy and chemotherapy on immunocompetence. A study of patients with acute myeloblastic leukemia in remission. Cancer Immunol. Immunother. (1978) (in press)
72. Vogler, W. R., Chan, Y. K.: Prolonging remission in myeloblastic leukaemia by tice-strain bacillus Calmette-Guérin. Lancet *1974 II*, 128–131
73. Vogler, W. R., Bartolucci, A. A., Omura, G. A., Miller, D., Smalley, R., Knopse, W. H., Goldstein, A.: A randomized clinical trial of BCG in myeloblastic leukemia conducted by the Southeastern Cancer Study Group. In: Immunotherapy of cancer: present status of trials in man. Terry, W. D., Windhorst, D. (eds.), pp. 365–373. New York: Raven Press 1978
74. Wanebo, H. J., Hilal, E., Strong, E. W., Pinsky, C., Oettgen, H. F., Hirshaut, Y.: Randomized trial of levamisole in patients with squamous cell carcinoma of the head and neck. In: Immune modulation and control of neoplasia by adjuvant therapy. Chirigos, M. A. (ed.). Cancer Treat. Rep. (1978) (in press)
75. Whittaker, J. A., Slater, A. J.: The immunotherapy of acute myelogenous leukaemia using intravenous BCG. In: Immunotherapy of cancer: present status of trials in man. Terry, W. D., Windhorst, D. (eds), pp. 393–404. New York: Raven Press 1978

Recent Results in Cancer Research

Sponsored by the Swiss League against Cancer. Editor in Chief: P. Rentchnick, Genève

For information about Vols. 1–9, please contact your bookseller or Springer-Verlag

10 NELSON, R. S.: Radioactive Phosphorus in the Diagnosis of Gastrointestinal Cancer.
11 FREEMAN, R. G. and J. M. KNOX: Treatment of Skin Cancer.
12 LYNCH, H. T.: Hereditary Factors in Carcinoma.
13 Tumours in Children, 2nd Edition. Edited by H. B. MARSDEN and J. K. STEWARD.
14 ODARTCHENKO, N.: Production Cellulaire Erythropoïétique.
15 SOKOLOFF, B.: Carcinoid and Serotonin.
16 JACOBS, M. L.: Malignant Lymphomas and Their Management.
17 Normal and Malignant Cell Growth. Edited by R. J. M. FRY, M. L. GRIEM, and W. H. KIRSTEN (Symposium).
18 ANGLESIO, E.: The Treatment of Hodgkin's Disease.
19 BANNASCH, P.: The Cytoplasm of Hepatocytes during Carcinogenesis. Electron- and Lightmicroscopical Investigations of the Nitrosomorpholineintoxicated Rat Liver.
20 Rubidomycin. A new Agent against Cancer. Edited by J. BERNARD, R. PAUL, M. BOIRON, C. JACQUILLAT, and R. MARAL.
21 Scientific Basis of Cancer Chemotherapy. Edited by G. MATHÉ (Symposium).
22 KOLDOVSKÝ, P.: Tumor Specific Transplantation Antigen.
23 FUCHS, W. A., J. W. Davidson, and H. W. FISCHER: Lymphography in Cancer. With contributions by G. JANTET and H. RÖSLER.
24 HAYWARD, J.: Hormones und Human Breast Cancer. An Account of 15 Years Study.
25 ROY-BURMAN, P.: Analogues of Nucleic Acid Components. Mechanisms of Action.
26 Tumors of the Liver. Edited by G. T. PACK and A. H. ISLAMI.
27 SZYMENDERA, J.: Bone Mineral Metabolism in Cancer.
28 MEEK, E. S.: Antitumour and Antiviral Substances of Natural Origin.
29 Aseptic Environments and Cancer Treatment. Edited by G. MATHÉ (Symposium).
30 Advances in the Treatment of Acute (Blastic) Leukemias. Edited by G. MATHÉ (Symposium).
31 DENOIX, P.: Treatment of Malignant Breast Tumors. Indications and Results.
32 NELSON, R. S.: Endoscopy in Gastric Cancer.
33 Experimental and Clinical Effects of L-Asparaginase. Edited by E. GRUNDMANN and H. F. OETTGEN (Symposium).
34 Chemistry and Biological Actions of 4-Nitroquinolin 1-Oxide. Edited by H. ENDO, T. ONO, and T. SUGIMURA.
35 PENN, I.: Malignant Tumors in Organ Transplant Recipients.
36 Current Concepts in the Management of Lymphoma and Leukemia. Edited by J. E. ULTMANN, M. L. GRIEM, W. H. KIRSTEN, and R. W. WISSLER (Symposium).
37 CHIAPPA, S., R. MUSUMECI, and C. USLENGHI: Endolymphatic Radiotherapy in Malignant Lymphomas. With contributions by G. BONADONNA, B. DAMASCELLI, G. FAVA, F. PIZZETTI, U. VERONESI.
38 KOLLER, P. C.: The Role of Chromosomes in Cancer Biology.
39 Current Problems in the Epidemiology of Cancer and Lymphomas. Edited by E. GRUNDMANN and H. TULINIUS (Symposium).
40 LANGLEY, F. A. and A. C. CROMPTON: Epithelial Abnormalities of the Cervix Uteri.
41 Tumours in a Tropical Country. A Survey of Uganda (1964–1968). Edited by A. C. TEMPLETON.
42 Breast Cancer: A Challenging Problem. Edited by M. L. GRIEM, E. V. JENSEN, J. E. ULTMANN, and R. W. WISSLER (Symposium).
43 Nomenclature, Methodology and Results of Clinical Trials in Acute Leukemias. Edited by G. MATHÉ, P. POUILLART, L. SCHWARZENBERG (Symposium).
44 Special Topics in Carcinogenesis. Edited by E. GRUNDMANN (Symposium).
45 KOLDOVSKÝ, P.: Carcinoembryonic Antigens.
46 Diagnosis and Therapy of Malignant Lymphoma. Edited by K. MUSSHOFF (Symposium).
47 Investigation and Stimulation of Immunity in Cancer Patients. Edited by G. MATHÉ and R. WEINER (Symposium).
48 Platinum Coordination Complexes in Cancer Chemotherapy. Edited by T. A. CONNORS and J. J. ROBERTS (Symposium).
49 Complications of Cancer Chemotherapy. Edited by G. MATHÉ and R. K. OLDHAM (Symposium).
50 Cancer Registry, Edited by E. GRUNDMANN and E. PEDERSEN (Symposium).

51 Gliomas. Current Concepts in Biology, Diagnosis and Therapy. Edited by J. HEKMATPANAH (Symposium).

52 The Ambivalence of Cytostatic Therapy. Edited by E. GRUNDMANN and R. GROSS (Symposium).

53 A. CLARYSSE, Y. KENIS, and G. MATHÉ: Cancer Chemotherapy.

54 Malignant Bone Tumors. Edited by E. GRUNDMANN.

55 MATHÉ, G.: Cancer Active Immunotherapy, Immunoprophylaxis, and Immunorestoration.

56 Lymphocytes, Macrophages, and Cancer. Edited by G. MATHÉ, I. FLORENTIN, and M.-C. SIMMLER (Symposium).

57 Breast Cancer: A Multidisciplinary Approach. Edited by G. ST. ARNEAULT, P. BAND, and L. ISRAËL (Symposium).

58 B. S. SCHOENBERG: Multiple Primary Malignant Neoplasms.

59 Selective Heat Sensitivity of Cancer Cells. Edited by A. ROSSI-FANELLI, R. CAVALIERE, B. MONDOVI, and G. MORICCA.

60 Tumors of the Male Genital System. Edited by E. GRUNDMANN and W. VAHLENSIECK (Symposium).

61 D. METCALF: Hemopoietic Colonies.

62 Tactics and Strategy in Cancer Treatment. Edited by G. MATHÉ (Symposium).

63 Antitumor Antibiotics. Edited by S. K. CARTER, H. UMEZAWA, J. DOUROS, and Y. SAKURAI (Symposium).

64 Lymphoid Neoplasias I: Classification, Categorization, Natural History.

65 Lymphoid Neoplasias II: Clinical and Therapeutic Aspects.
Lymphoid Neoplasias I & II. Proceedings of the 1977 CNRS-EORTC International Colloquium. Editors: G. MATHÉ, M. SELIGMANN, M. TUBIANA. Devided into two volumes.

66 Carcinogenic Hormones. Edited by C. H. LINGEMAN.

67/68 Adjuvant Therapies and Markers of Post-Surgical Minimal Residual Disease I & II. Proceedings of the 1978 Annual Plenary Meeting of the EORTC. Editors: G. BONADONNA, G. MATHÉ, S. E. SALMON. Divided into two volumes:

67 Markers and General Problems of Cancer Adjuvant Therapies.

68 Adjuvant Therapies and Markers of the Various Primary Tumors.

MIX
Papier aus verantwortungsvollen Quellen
Paper from responsible sources
FSC® C105338

If you have any concerns about our products,
you can contact us on
ProductSafety@springernature.com

In case Publisher is established outside the EU,
the EU authorized representative is:
Springer Nature Customer Service Center GmbH
Europaplatz 3, 69115 Heidelberg, Germany

Printed by Libri Plureos GmbH
in Hamburg, Germany